Springer Series: THE TEACHING OF NURSING

Series Editor: Diane McGivern, RN, PhD, FAAN

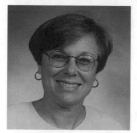 **Marilyn Oermann, PhD, RN, FAAN** is a Professor in the College of Nursing at Wayne State University, Detroit, MI. She is the author of seven books and many articles on clinical teaching, clinical evaluation, and teaching strategies in nursing education. She has presented workshops, conferences, and speeches on teaching and evaluation in nursing.

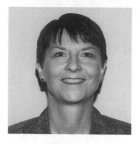 **Kathleen B. Gaberson, PhD, RN,** is an Associate Professor at Duquesne University School of Nursing in Pittsburgh, PA, where she teaches courses in evaluation in nursing education and measurement issues in nursing research at the master's and doctoral levels. She has over 25 years of teaching experience in graduate, baccalaureate, diploma, staff development, and continuing nursing education programs. She lectures, writes, and consults extensively on measurement, evaluation, and other nursing education topics.

Evaluation and Testing in Nursing Education

Marilyn H. Oermann,
PhD, RN, FAAN

Kathleen B. Gaberson,
PhD, RN

 Springer Series on the Teaching of Nursing

Springer Publishing Company, Inc.
536 Broadway
New York, NY 10012-3955

Acquisitions Editor: Ruth Chasek
Cover design by Margaret Dunin
Production Editor: Pamela Lankas

99 00 01 02 / 5 4 3 2

Library of Congress Cataloging-in-Publication Data

Oermann, Marilyn H.
    Evaluation and testing in nursing education / Marilyn H. Oermann. Kathleen B. Gaberson.
        p.   cm. — (Springer series on the teaching of nursing)
    Includes bibliograpical references and index.
    ISBN 0-8261-9950-X
    1. Nursing—Examinations. 2. Nursing—Ability testing. 3. Nursing—Study and teaching—Evaluation. I. Gaberson, Kathleen B. II. Title. III. Series: Springer series on the teaching of nursing (unnumbered)
    [DNLM: 1. Education, Nursing—standards—United States. 2. Educational Measurement—methods. 3. Evaluation Studies. WY 18 029a 1998]
    RT73.7.047   1998
    610.73'071'1—dc21
    DNLM/DLC
    for Library of Congress   97-42741
                                                                          CIP

Printed in the United States of America

In memory of Sr. Mary Albert Kramer, an expert teacher
who introduced us to the concepts of evaluation and testing
in nursing education.

This book is also dedicated to our families:
David, Eric, and Ross Oermann

Paul Gaberson and Matthew Ammon

Contents

Contributor

Chapter 16 entitled *Total Quality Management and Nursing Education* was written by:

Theresa L. Carroll, PhD, RN
Professor and Associate Dean for Academic Affairs
School of Nursing
University of Texas—Houston
Houston, Texas

Preface

At some time or another all teachers are faced with the need to measure and evaluate learning in a course, workshop, continuing education program, and following other types of instruction. As part of this measurement and evaluation process, the teacher may write test items, prepare tests and analyze their results, develop rating scales and other types of clinical evaluation methods, and plan other strategies for assessing learning in the classroom and practice setting.

Often teachers are not prepared to carry out these tasks as part of their instructional role. *Evaluation and Testing in Nursing Education* is a resource for teachers in schools of nursing and health care agencies; for students preparing for teaching roles; for nurses in practice who teach others and are therefore responsible for evaluating their learning; and for other health professionals involved in measurement, evaluation, and testing. Although the examples provided of test items and other types of evaluation methods are nursing oriented, they are easily adapted to other health fields.

The purposes of the book are to describe the concepts of measurement, evaluation, and testing in nursing education; to elucidate the qualities of effective measurement instruments; to detail how to plan for classroom testing, write test items, assemble and administer tests, and analyze test results; to offer strategies for evaluating critical thinking and other higher level cognitive skills; to illustrate the concepts of performance evaluation and how to assess clinical competencies; to outline the social, ethical, and legal issues associated with evaluation and testing; as well as to explain program evaluation and other related principles of measurement and evaluation. The content is useful for teachers in any setting who are involved in evaluating others, whether they be students, nurses, or other types of health personnel.

The book is organized into five broad areas: (a) concepts of measurement, evaluation, and testing; (b) test construction and analyzing tests; (c) clinical and performance evaluation; (d) interpreting and reporting test results; and (e) evaluating educational programs. Each chapter contains an in-depth discussion of the content accompanied by examples to make the principles clear to the reader.

The first section of the book contains two chapters; chapter 1 addresses the purposes of measurement and evaluation in nursing education and introduces important concepts that influence how teachers measure and evaluate learning in nursing. Differences between formative and summative evaluation and between norm- and criterion-referenced measurement are explored. Because effective evaluation requires a clear description of *what* and *how* to evaluate, the chapter describes the use of objectives as a basis for developing test items and evaluation strategies, provides examples of objectives at different taxonomic levels, and describes how test items would be developed at each of these levels.

In chapter 2 qualities of effective measurement instruments are discussed. The concepts of validity and reliability and their effects on the interpretive quality of measurement results are described in the chapter. To make judgments about the valid use of a set of scores, teachers must gather one or more types of validity evidence: content-related, criterion-related, and construct-related; each of these types is discussed in chapter 2. Different types of reliability also are explained and examples provided. Also discussed in chapter 2 are important practical considerations that might affect the choice or development of tests and other instruments.

Chapters in the second section of the book revolve around test construction and analyzing tests. Chapter 3 discusses the steps involved in planning for test construction, enabling the teacher to make good decisions about what and when to test, test length, difficulty of test items, item formats, and scoring procedures. An important focus of the chapter is how to develop a test blueprint and then use it for writing test items; different examples are provided to clarify this process for the reader. Broad principles important in developing test items, regardless of the specific type, are described in the chapter.

Chapters 4 through 7 discuss all types of test items, beginning with objective-type items, progressing to essay and written assignments, and ending with evaluating critical thinking and higher level cognitive skills. Chapter 4 discusses initially how to decide on the type of test item and other evaluation strategy to use; advantages and disadvantages of objective-type items compared with other formats are explored in the chapter. Three types of objective test items are then presented: true–false and different variations of true–false items, matching exercises, and short answer. Principles for writing each type of item are presented accompanied by sample items.

An entire chapter, 5, is devoted to developing multiple-choice items, considering that this is the predominant format used for testing in nursing not only in terms of teacher-made tests but also for licensing, certification, and other commercially available examinations. There is extensive discussion of how to write the stem, answer, and distracters for a multiple-choice item. Principles to be followed in developing multiple-choice items are explained in the chapter, and examples are provided to illustrate them. A section is included on writing multiple-choice items about phases of the nursing process and decisions to be made in a clinical situation that require application of concepts and theories to arrive at an answer. The relationship of these items to the NCLEX is discussed. A brief description of multiple-response items also is included in chapter 5.

Chapter 6 shifts from objective-type items to writing and evaluating essay items and written assignments. Discussion includes suggestions for preparing restricted- and extended-response essay items, the reliability of essay tests, and suggestions for scoring items including the holistic and analytical methods. Chapter 6 also describes how to evaluate written assignments.

There is much discussion in nursing, among students and nurses alike, about development of critical-thinking ability. Chapter 7 focuses on evaluating problem-solving, decision-making, and critical-thinking skills. Context-dependent item sets are discussed as one format of testing appropriate for assessing higher level cognitive skills. Suggestions for developing them are presented in the chapter, including examples illustrating the cognitive ability being examined by the item. Other evaluation strategies also are described: case method and case study, discussion questions for higher level thinking and Socratic questioning, debate, media clips, and short written assignments for evaluating critical thinking. Standardized instruments for measuring critical thinking are reviewed in the chapter.

Chapter 8 explains how to assemble and administer a test. In addition to preparing a test blueprint and skillful construction of test items, the final appearance of the test and way in which it is administered can affect the validity of its results. In chapter 8, test design rules are described; suggestions for reproducing the test, maintaining test security, administering it, and preventing cheating are also presented in the chapter.

After administering the test, it needs to be scored, results interpreted, and then used to make varied decisions. Chapter 9 discusses the processes of obtaining scores and performing test and item analysis. It also suggests ways in which teachers can use posttest discussions to contribute to student learning and seek student feedback that can lead to test item improvement. The chapter begins with a discussion of scoring tests, including weighting items and correction for guessing, then proceeds to item analysis. How to calculate the difficulty index and discrimination index and analyze each distracter are described; performing an item analysis by hand is explained with an illustration for teachers who do not have computer software for this purpose. A section of the chapter also presents suggestions and examples of developing a test item bank.

The third section of the book explores evaluation in the clinical setting, an important dimension of evaluation in nursing and other health professions. Chapter 10 describes principles of clinical evaluation, the concept of fairness in evaluation, the stress experienced by learners in clinical practice and its relationship to evaluation, incorporating feedback within the evaluation process, and what to evaluate—establishing the clinical objectives or competencies.

Building on this discussion, chapter 11 presents methods for clinical evaluation: observation and recording observations in anecdotal notes, checklists, and rating scales; simulations and games for formative evaluation; media clips; written assignments accompanying the clinical experience, including journal writing; portfolio assessment and how to set up a portfolio system for clinical evaluation; conferences; clinical examination; and self-evaluation. Discussion includes the many types of rating scales used in nursing, errors that may occur in rating clinical performance, and how to avoid them.

Chapters 12 to 14 comprise the fourth section of the book on interpreting and reporting test results. In chapter 12, the discussion focuses on how to interpret the meaning of test scores. Basic statistical concepts are presented and used for criterion- and norm-referenced interpretations of teacher-made and standardized test results.

Chapter 13 examines the purposes of grades, criticisms of grades, types of grading systems, assigning letter grades, selecting a grading framework, and how to calculate grades with each of these frameworks. Once again, examples are provided to illustrate these principles for the reader. A section of the chapter is devoted to grading clinical practice, pass-fail and other systems for grading, and suggestions for the teacher when students have the potential for failing clinical practice. Legal principles are integrated within this discussion.

Chapter 14 explores social, ethical, and legal issues associated with testing and evaluation. Social issues such as test bias, grade inflation, and effects of testing on self-esteem are discussed. Ethical issues include privacy and access to test results; strategies for preventing legal problems are explored in the chapter.

Chapters 15 and 16 conclude the book by forming the final section on evaluating educational programs and teachers. Chapter 15 examines broad principles of program and teacher evaluation, and chapter 16 introduces the reader to total quality management and nursing education.

The authors wish to acknowledge some of the many people who contributed to the preparation of this book. Susan Housholder, MSN, CCRN and Maria Teresa Palleschi, MSN, CCRN reviewed the test items in the book; Janet P. Zinn, MSN, developed and reviewed selected test items for chapter 5. Joanne Turka, MSN, developed one of the clinical evaluation instruments in Appendix A. We are thankful for supportive families who assumed many additional responsibilities during the writing of the book: David, Ross, and Eric Oermann, Paul Gaberson, and Matthew Ammon.

Marilyn Oermann
Kathy Gaberson

1

Evaluation, Measurement, and the Educational Process

I n all areas of nursing education and practice, evaluation is an important process used to measure learning and health-related outcomes,
monitor performance, determine competence to practice, and arrive at
other decisions about individuals and organizations. Evaluation is integral
to monitoring the quality of educational and health care programs.
Important decisions often rest on evaluation, and all educators regardless
of the setting need to be knowledgeable about the evaluation process, measurement, testing, assessment, and other related concepts.

In nursing education and practice today, there is increasing emphasis
on evaluation, with nursing programs and institutions determining the
outcomes achieved by students, graduates, and clients as one indicator of
the effectiveness of their programs. Evaluation also provides a means of
ensuring accountability for the quality of education and services provided.
Nursing, similar to other professions, is accountable to the clients served
and to society in general for meeting their health needs. Along the same
line, nurse educators are accountable for the quality of teaching provided
to learners, outcomes achieved, and overall effectiveness of programs that
prepare graduates to meet the health needs of society. Educational institutions also are accountable to their governing bodies and society in terms
of educating graduates for present and future roles. Evaluation is important in answering questions about our accountability for quality educational programs and health care services.

EVALUATION

Evaluation is the process of obtaining information for making judgments about the quality of student learning or achievement, clinical performance, employee competence, and educational programs. In nursing education evaluation typically takes the form of judging student attainment of educational objectives and goals in the classroom and the quality of student performance in the clinical setting. The student's educational experiences result in changes in the learner; evaluation provides the means of assessing these changes. With this evaluation, learning outcomes are measured, further educational needs are identified, and additional instruction can be planned to move the student toward attainment of the learning objectives and development of essential competencies for practice. Similarly, evaluation of employees provides information on their performance at varied points in time.

In terms of educational programs, evaluation includes collecting information at three points of the process: prior to developing the program, during the process of program development to provide a basis for ongoing revision, and after implementing the program to determine its effectiveness. Bevil (1991) defines program evaluation as the systematic and continuous process of gathering and analyzing data about all dimensions of the program and then using this information for decision making about program quality and effectiveness (p. 60). Faculty are involved in program evaluation as they revise their programs and measure outcomes for accreditation and other purposes. While many of the concepts described in this book are applicable to program evaluation, the focus here is on evaluating learners, whether they be students in a nursing program or nurses in a health care setting. The term "students" is used broadly to incorporate both of these groups of learners.

Evaluation is the process of making value judgments about learners; value, in fact, is part of the word *evaluation*. Ebel and Frisbie (1991) suggested that these questions of value require judgment by the teacher, making evaluation a complex and difficult process. Value judgments about the desirability of the results, answering the question "how good?," are a significant part of the evaluation process (Gronlund & Linn, 1990). As teachers carry out evaluation, their own values and beliefs influence the process. Faculty who value speed in clinical practice, for instance, may find that their judgments about students are influenced by this value, regardless of the objective or outcome being evaluated. The nature of evaluation suggests that teachers need to assess their own values and beliefs as they may influence the data collected and judgments made about students. Tanner (1994) proposed that professional judgments are "at the heart" of effective

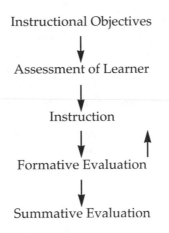

Figure 1.1 Relationship between instruction and evalution.

Note. From *Clinical Teaching in Nursing Education* (2nd ed., p. 152), by D. E. Reilly and M. H. Oermann, 1992. New York. National League for Nursing. Copyright 1992 by National League for Nursing. Reprinted with permission.

evaluations; clear and reasonable standards of performance are needed against which to base these judgments. Regardless of the specificity of the standards and criteria used for evaluating learners, evaluation remains a subjective process (Orchard, 1994; Reilly & Oermann, 1992; Tanner, 1994).

Evaluation is the systematic process of collecting and interpreting information as a basis for decisions about learners. Through evaluation the teacher determines the progress of students toward meeting the educational objectives and developing competencies and their achievement of them; evaluation is a continuing, open-ended process closely interwoven with teaching and learning (Reilly & Oermann, 1990, 1992). Evaluation provides information about learner progress that forms a basis for further instruction. Figure 1.1 demonstrates the relationship between evaluation and the instructional process. The educational objectives specify the intended learning outcomes whether they be for classroom attainment, clinical practice, or learning in other settings. Following assessment of learner needs in terms of these objectives, the teacher plans and delivers the instruction. This instructional component includes developing the plan for learning, developing educational materials and activities, selecting learning experiences, and teaching learners in varied settings.

The remaining components of the instructional process relate to evaluation. The first evaluation component, formative evaluation, deals with evaluating student progress toward meeting the objectives and demonstrating competency in clinical practice. This type of evaluation is displayed with a feedback loop to instruction, for formative evaluation provides information about further learning needs of students and where additional instruction is needed. In summative evaluation, the focus is at the end of instruction to determine if the objectives have been achieved and competencies developed. Bott (1996) would add a final component to the instructional process, evaluating the effectiveness of the teacher. He emphasized that evaluation of student performance and teacher effectiveness provide information for reteaching, reassessing, and redesigning the objectives, emphasizing the cyclical nature of the instructional process.

Formative Evaluation

Evaluation fulfills two major roles in the classroom and clinical setting: formative and summative. A third role of evaluation, confirmative, reflects continuing evaluation of learner competence at some point after summative evaluation. Formative evaluation reflects feedback to learners about their progress in meeting the objectives and developing competencies for practice. It occurs throughout the instructional process and provides a basis for determining where further learning is needed. As such, formative evaluation is diagnostic, providing information to the teacher and learner about the progress being made in meeting the objectives.

In the classroom, formative information may be collected by teacher observation and questioning of students, diagnostic quizzes, and in- and out-of-class assignments. In clinical practice, formative evaluation is an integral part of the instructional process. The teacher continually makes observations of and questions the learner, reviews and provides feedback on documentation and student clinical assignments, evaluates student decisions regarding the planning and implementation of care, and arrives at judgments about student progress in acquiring essential clinical knowledge and skills for care of clients. The teacher's role is critical to provide feedback to learners about their progress in achieving the goals of clinical practice.

Considering that the purpose of formative evaluation is to provide feedback on the progress being made in learning, typically, formative evaluation is not graded. Gronlund and Linn (1990) stated that "Since formative evaluation is directed toward improving learning and instruction, the results are typically *not* used for assigning course grades" (p. 13). It is important for the teacher to remember that the purpose of formative evaluation is to assess where further learning is needed.

Summative Evaluation

Summative evaluation, on the other hand, is end-of-instruction evaluation designed to determine what the student has learned in the classroom and clinical setting. Summative evaluation provides information on the extent to which objectives were achieved, not on the progress of the learner in meeting them. As such, summative evaluation occurs at the end of the learning process, for instance, at the end of a course, to determine the student's grade and certify competence. While formative evaluation occurs throughout the learning experience, for example, daily, summative evaluation is conducted on a periodic basis, for instance, every few weeks, or at the midterm and final evaluation periods. This type of evaluation is "final" in nature and serves as a basis for grading student achievement.

Summative evaluation assesses typically broader content areas than does formative evaluation, which tends to be more specific in terms of the content evaluated. Methods commonly used for summative evaluation in the classroom include tests, term papers, and other types of projects. In clinical practice, written assignments, projects completed about clinical experiences, rating scales, and other performance measures may be used. Both formative and summative evaluation are essential components of most nursing courses.

Confirmative Evaluation

Another role of evaluation is confirmative. The purpose of confirmative evaluation is to collect, examine, and interpret data to determine the continuing competence of learners, thereby allowing the teacher to assess if learners remain competent (Hellebrandt & Russell, 1993). The notion of confirmative evaluation is significant in the health professions in terms of assuring that learners maintain their clinical knowledge and skills. Confirmative evaluation takes place after completion of the instruction, for instance, following development of skills in the learning laboratory or clinical setting, "to decide if the competencies are still satisfactory or if the learner needs to undergo additional instruction" (Hellebrandt & Russell, 1993, p. 26). With this follow-up evaluation of clinical competencies, after summative evaluation, the teacher can identify which students need further practice of skills. Confirmative evaluation in nursing is significant, particularly in the clinical setting, to assure that learners maintain their competencies and to identify where additional review and practice are needed. Confirmative evaluation is conducted typically through observations, ratings scales, and use of performance checklists in the clinical setting or learning laboratory. Faculty may set up simulations to serve this purpose.

MEASUREMENT

Measurement is the process of assigning numbers to represent student achievement according to certain rules. It answers the question "How much?" Gronlund and Linn (1990) emphasized that measurement is limited to quantitative descriptions of students, expressing their achievement in numbers, for instance, answering 85 out of 100 items correctly on a test. Measurement, in contrast to evaluation, does not imply value judgments about the quality of the results. Measurement is important for describing the achievement of learners on nursing and other tests, but not all outcomes important in nursing practice can be measured by testing. Many outcomes are evaluated qualitatively through other means, such as observations of performance.

Although measurement results in assigning numbers to reflect learning, these numbers in and of themselves have no meaning. Scoring 15 on a test means nothing unless it is referenced or compared with other students' scores or to a predetermined standard. Perhaps 15 was the highest or lowest score on the test compared with other students. Or, the student might have set a personal goal of achieving 15 on the test, and meeting this goal is more important than how others scored on the test. Another interpretation is that a score of 15 might reflect the standard expected of this particular group of learners. Having a reference point with which to compare a particular test score is essential to give it meaning, to interpret the score.

In clinical practice, how does a learner's performance compare with that of others in the group? Does the learner meet the clinical objectives and possess certain competencies, regardless of how other students in the group perform in clinical practice? Answers to these questions depend on the basis used for interpreting performance similar to interpreting the test scores described earlier.

Norm-Referenced Measurement

There are two main ways of interpreting test scores and other types of evaluation conducted in the clinical setting: norm- and-criterion referenced. In norm-referenced measurement, test scores and other evaluation data are referenced to a norm group. Norm-referenced interpretation compares a student's test scores with others in the class or with some other group. The student's score may be described as below or above average or at a certain rank in the class. Norm-referenced clinical evaluation compares students' clinical performance with that of a group of learners, indicating that the learner has more or less clinical competence than others in the group. A clinical evaluation instrument in which student performance is rated on a scale of below to above average reflects a norm-referenced system.

Criterion-Referenced Measurement

Criterion-referenced measurement, on the other hand, involves interpreting scores based on preset criteria, not in relation to the group of learners. With this type of measurement, an individual score is compared to a preset standard or criterion. The concern is how well the student performs and what the student can do, but not in comparison with other students in the group. Gronlund and Linn (1990) described various criterion-referenced interpretations: (a) describing the specific learning tasks a student can perform, (b) indicating the percentage of tasks performed or items answered correctly, and (c) comparing test performance against a set standard (p. 14). Criterion-referenced testing determines how well the student performs at the end of the instruction in comparison with the behavior indicated in the course and instructional objectives (Bott, 1996).

With criterion-referenced clinical evaluation, student performance is compared with a set of criteria to be met. The clinical objectives and other statements of competencies to be performed in clinical practice are examples of these criteria. In clinical practice, student performance is measured against the criteria, the concern being whether or not students achieve the clinical objectives or meet the competencies, and not how well they perform in comparison to others.

TESTING

Tests are one form of measurement. A test is a set of questions, each with a correct answer, to which the student responds in written form or orally (Ebel & Frisbie, 1991, p. 26). Tests, then, are a type of measurement tool. Bott (1996) emphasized that tests are an indirect measure of achievement; learning is assumed to have occurred when students score at a particular level on the test.

While students in all fields often dread tests, information provided from tests enables faculty to make important decisions regarding the instruction. Kubiszyn and Borich (1993) identified a number of these decisions relevant to nursing programs:

1. *Instructional*, enabling the teacher to identify content areas learned effectively by students and ones requiring further instruction;

2. *Grading,* for which tests serve typically as one type of data;
3. *Diagnostic,* to identify the student's strengths and weaknesses;
4. *Selection,* using test data to accept or reject applicants to nursing programs;
5. *Placement,* after the individual has been admitted to the program, such as placement testing for registered nurses;
6. *Counseling,* involving the use of test data to recommend appropriate programs of study for the student; and
7. *Program and curriculum,* using test data as one source of information for program and curriculum evaluation.

ASSESSMENT

Although a test is a one-time measure, assessment involves the collection of data about learners and programs over a period of time. Mitchell (1992) indicated that the purpose of assessment is to examine the quality of a student's work or educational program extending over time. Assessment involves techniques such as student portfolios, open-ended questions, observations, and projects (Mitchell, 1992). In nursing education, much discussion has involved the assessment of learning outcomes. Keith (1991) described this process as first stating clearly the learning outcomes, what students should learn and be able to do at the end of a program of study, then using assessment to provide information about the extent of their achievement (p. 1).

OBJECTIVES FOR EVALUATION AND MEASUREMENT

Instructional objectives play an important role in teaching students in varied settings in nursing. They provide guidelines for student learning and instruction and the basis for evaluating learning. The objectives represent the outcomes of learning; these outcomes may include the acquisition of knowledge, development of values, and performance of psychomotor and technological skills. Evaluation serves to determine the extent of the student's learning in relation to these outcomes. This does not mean that the teacher is unconcerned about learning that occurs and is not expressed as objectives. It is anticipated that many students will acquire knowledge, values, and skills beyond those expressed in the objectives. Learning beyond the objectives does occur and should be reflected in the evaluation protocol (Reilly & Oermann, 1990).

Gronlund and Linn (1990) emphasized that effective evaluation requires a clear description of *what* to evaluate and *how* to evaluate it. Before developing tests, planning clinical evaluation methods, and designing other evaluation measures, the teacher needs to specify clearly the intended learning outcomes (p. 24).

Writing Objectives

In developing instructional objectives, there are two important dimensions to consider. The first is the actual technique for writing objectives, the second is ordering their complexity based on the taxonomies. There are different formats for writing objectives. One type results in a highly specific objective that includes a description of the learner, behaviors the learner will exhibit at the end of the instruction, conditions under which the learner will demonstrate competence, and a standard of performance (Reilly & Oermann, 1990, p. 40). An example of a specific instructional objective is: Given a written nursing assessment, the student identifies in writing two nursing diagnoses with supporting rationale. This objective includes the following components:

Learner:	Student
Behavior:	Identifies in writing nursing diagnoses
Conditions:	Given a written nursing assessment
Standard:	Two nursing diagnoses must be identified with supporting rationale

It is clear from the example that this type of objective is prescriptive and provides minimal flexibility for both teacher and student. The complexity of learning expected in nursing makes it difficult to use such a system for specifying the objectives. With this specificity, faculty would need numerous objectives to indicate the outcomes of learning for a course. For these reasons, a general format for writing objectives is sufficient to express the learning outcomes and provide a basis for evaluating learning.

General objectives include a description of the learner, behavior the learner will exhibit at the end of the instruction, and content to which the behavior relates. A general objective similar to the earlier outcome is: The student identifies nursing diagnoses from the assessment. With this example, the components would be:

Learner:	Student
Behavior:	Identifies
Content:	Nursing diagnoses from the assessment

This general objective, which is open-ended, provides flexibility for the teacher in developing instruction to meet it and for evaluating student learning. The outcome could be met and evaluated in the classroom through varied activities in which students analyze assessment data—presented orally, in written form, or through multimedia—and identify nursing diagnoses. Students might work in groups in the learning laboratory reviewing various assessments and completing simulations to identify nursing diagnoses. In the clinical setting patient assignments, conferences, discussions with students, and review of patient records provide other strategies for developing the ability to derive nursing diagnoses and for evaluating student competency. Generally stated objectives, therefore, provide sufficient guidelines for instruction and evaluation of student learning. For these reasons, only generally stated objectives are used as examples in the book.

The objectives are important in developing evaluation methods which measure the behavior and content area intended by the objective. In evaluating the above objective, the method selected, for instance, a test, needs to examine student ability to identify nursing diagnoses from assessment data. The objective does not specify the number of nursing diagnoses, type of client problem, complexity of the assessment data, or other variables associated with the clinical situation; there is opportunity for teachers to develop various types of test questions and evaluation measures as long as they ask the learner to identify nursing diagnoses based on the given assessment.

Ebel and Frisbie (1991) indicated that clearly written objectives guide the teacher in selecting evaluation methods. The behavior indicated by the objective suggests an evaluation method, such as tests, observations in the clinical setting, papers, and others. When tests are chosen as the method, the objective in turn suggests the type of test question, for instance, true-false, multiple-choice, and essay.

In addition to guiding decisions about evaluation methods, the objective gives clues to faculty about teaching methods and learning activities to assist students in meeting it. For the sample objective, teaching methods might include: readings, lecture, discussion, case study, simulation, videotape, computer-assisted instruction, interactive video, role play, clinical practice, conference, and other methods that present assessment data and ask students to identify varied nursing diagnoses.

Techniques for writing objectives have been described elsewhere in the literature. Important points in writing objectives to provide an adequate basis for designing the evaluation include:

1. *The behavior, or action verb, should be specific and measurable.* It represents the outcome expected of the learner at the end of the instruction.

Table 1.1 Sample Behaviors Appropriate for Each Taxonomic Level

Cognitive domain	Affective domain	Psychomotor domain
Knowledge	Receiving	Imitation
Define	Acknowledge	Follow example of
Identify	Show awareness of	Imitate
List		
Name	Responding	Manipulation
Recall	Acts willingly	Carry out according
	Is willing to support	to procedure
Comprehension	Respond	Follow procedure
Demonstrate use of	Seek opportunities	Practice following
Describe		procedure
Differentiate	Valuing	
Draw conclusions	Accept	Precision
Explain	Assume responsibility	Demonstrate skill
Give examples of	Participate in	Is accurate in
Interpret	Respect	
Select	Support	Articulation
	Value	Carry out accurately
Application		and in reasonable
Apply	Organization of values	time frame
Relate	Argue	Is skillful
Use	Debate	
	Declare	Naturalization
Analysis	Defend	Is competent
Analyze	Take a stand	Carry out compe-
Compare		tently
Contrast	Characterization by value	Integrate skill within
Detect	Act consistently	care
Identify	Stand for	
Relate		
Synthesis		
Construct		
Design		
Develop		
Produce		
Synthesize		
Evaluation		
Appraise		
Assess		
Critique		
Evaluate		
Judge		

Note. From *Behavioral Objectives: Evaluation in Nursing* (3rd ed., pp. 85–86), by D. E. Reilly and M. H. Oermann, 1990, New York: National League for Nursing. Copyright 1990 by National League for Nursing. Adapted with permission.

Terms such as "identify," "describe," and "analyze" are specific and may be measured; words such as "understand" and "know," in contrast, represent a wide variety of behaviors, some simple and others complex, making these terms difficult to evaluate. The student's knowledge might range from identifying and naming through synthesizing and evaluating. Sample behaviors are presented in Table 1.1.

2. *Include one behavior per objective.* If more than one behavior is included in the objective, instances may arise in which students achieve only one of the behaviors, limiting decisions as to whether or not they met the objective.

3. *Keep the objectives as general as possible* to allow for their achievement with varied course content. For instance, instead of stating that "the student identifies physiological nursing diagnoses from the assessment of acutely ill patients," indicating that "the learner identifies nursing diagnoses from assessment data" provides more flexibility for the teacher in designing evaluation strategies which reflect different types of diagnoses from varied data sets presented in the course. Gronlund and Linn (1990) referred to this form of objective as content-free; the objectives can be used with various units of study and provide a wider range of course material for testing (p. 40).

4. *Omit stating the teaching method in the objective* to provide greater flexibility in how the objective is taught and evaluated. For instance, in the following objective, the teacher is limited to evaluating communication techniques through simulations rather than interactions the student might have in the clinical setting: The learner uses effective communication techniques in a simulated client–nurse interaction. The objective might be stated more broadly as: The learner uses effective communication techniques with clients.

Taxonomies of Educational Objectives

The need for clearly stated objectives becomes evident when the teacher translates them into test items and other evaluation methods. Test items need to adequately measure the behavior in the objective, for instance, identify, describe, apply, and analyze, as it relates to the content area. Objectives may be written to reflect three domains of learning, each with its own classification or taxonomic system: cognitive, affective, and psychomotor.

A taxonomy is a classification system which places an objective within a broader system or scheme. While learning in nursing ultimately represents an integration of these domains, it is valuable in planning instruction, and particularly in developing evaluation measures, for the domains to be considered separately.

COGNITIVE DOMAIN

The cognitive domain deals with knowledge and intellectual skills. Learning within this domain includes the acquisition of facts and specific information underlying the practice of nursing; concepts, theories, and principles about nursing; and cognitive skills such as decision-making, problem-solving, clinical judgment, and critical thinking. The cognitive taxonomy was developed by Bloom, Englehart, Furst, Hill, and Krathwohl in 1956. It provides for six levels of cognitive learning, increasing in complexity: knowledge, comprehension, application, analysis, synthesis, and evaluation. This hierarchy suggests that knowledge, such as recall of specific facts, is less intellectually complex and demanding than the higher levels of learning. Evaluation, the most complex level, requires judgments based on varied criteria. Bloom et al. (1956) identified sublevels for every level except "application."

Ebel and Frisbie (1991) suggested that one of the reasons the cognitive domain has received the most attention from test developers is that it creates an awareness as to the level of learning intended in the objective and to be evaluated. Teachers who expect application of knowledge can use the taxonomy to gear their objectives and evaluation methods to this level, rather than focusing only on the recall of facts and other information. If the teacher intends a higher level of learning as the outcome, then test items and other evaluation strategies also need to reflect this level.

In using the taxonomy, the teacher decides first on the level of cognitive learning intended and then develops objectives and evaluation methods for that particular level. The decision as to the taxonomic level at which to gear instruction and evaluation depends on the teacher's judgment considering the background of the learner (Reilly & Oermann, 1990); placement of the course and learning experiences within the curriculum to provide for the progressive development of knowledge, skills, and values; and complexity of the behavior and content in relation to the time allowed for teaching. If the time for teaching and evaluation is limited, the objectives may be written at a lower level. The taxonomy provides a continuum for educators to use in planning instruction and carrying out evaluation, beginning with recall of facts and information and progressing toward understanding, using concepts and theories in practice, analyzing situations, synthesizing from different sources to develop new products, and evaluating materials and situations based on internal and external criteria.

A description and sample objective for each of the six levels of learning in the cognitive taxonomy follow. Although sublevels have been established for these levels, except for application, only the six major levels are essential to guide the teacher for instructional and evaluation purposes.

1. *Knowledge*: Recall of facts and specific information. Memorization of specifics.
   The student defines the term "systole."

2. *Comprehension:* Understanding. Ability to describe and explain the material.
   The learner describes the circulation through the heart.

3. *Application*: Use of information in a new situation. Ability to use knowledge in a new situation.
   The student applies concepts of aging in developing interventions for the elderly.

4. *Analysis*: Ability to break down material into component parts and identify the relationships among them.
   The student analyzes the organizational structure of the community health agency and its impact on client services.

5. *Synthesis*: Ability to develop a new product. Combining elements to form a new product.
   The student develops a plan for delivering services to elderly persons who are homebound.

6. *Evaluation*: Judgments about value based on internal and external criteria. Extent to which materials and objects meet criteria.
   The learner evaluates nursing research based on predetermined criteria.

Ebel and Frisbie (1991) indicated that while Bloom's taxonomy serves many purposes, it has limitations when used for classifying test items. It is difficult at times to classify test questions based on these taxonomic levels. A question written at the comprehension level may actually be at the knowledge level if students learned the content in class and only need to recall it to answer the item. Classifying a test question at the application level requires use of previously learned concepts and theories in a new situation. Whether or not the situation is novel for each student, however, is not known. Ebel and Frisbie (1991) pointed out that it is difficult to identify the "mental processes involved in answering a particular test question" which may alter the level of cognitive complexity of the item for each student (p. 52).

To compensate for this problem, Ebel (1965) developed a classification system designed for use in categorizing test questions, and not for the

Table 1.2 Comparison of Bloom's Taxonomy and Ebel's Guide for Categorizing Test Items

Bloom's Taxonomy	Ebel's Guide
Knowledge	Terminology
	Factual Information
Comprehension	Explanation
Application	Calculation
	Prediction
Analysis	
Synthesis	
Evaluation	Recommended actions
	Evaluation

purpose of writing objectives. Ebel's taxonomy has seven categories to classify test questions: Terminology, factual information, explanation, calculation, prediction, recommended action, and evaluation (Table 1.2). These are hierarchical, similar to Bloom's taxonomy, and provide a guide for faculty in developing test items along different levels of complexity, from simple questions dealing with content such as defining terms and recalling information, to more complex questions such as ones that ask students to plan nursing interventions, recommend actions to take with clients, and evaluate clinical situations.

AFFECTIVE DOMAIN

The affective domain relates to development of values, attitudes, and beliefs consistent with professional nursing practice. Developed by Krathwohl, Bloom, and Masia (1964), the taxonomy of the affective domain includes five levels organized hierarchically and based on the principle of increasing involvement of the learner and internalization of a value. Krathwohl et al. (1964) believed that objectives for learning could be specified in the affective domain and instruction provided to assist the learner in developing a value system that guides decisions and behaviors. The principle on which the affective taxonomy is based relates to the movement of the learner from mere awareness of a value, for instance, confidentiality, to internalization of that value as a basis for his or her own behavior.

There are two important dimensions in evaluating affective outcomes. The first relates to the student's knowledge of the values, attitudes, and beliefs which are important in guiding decisions in nursing. Prior to internalizing a value and using it as a basis for decision making and behavior, the student needs to know the values, attitudes, and beliefs that guide nursing practice. There is a cognitive base, therefore, to the development of a value system. Evaluation of this dimension focuses on student acquisition of knowledge about the values, attitudes, and beliefs consistent with professional nursing practice. A variety of test questions and evaluation methods are appropriate to assess this knowledge base. The second dimension of affective evaluation focuses on whether or not students have accepted these values, attitudes, and beliefs and are internalizing them to form a system for their own decision making and behavior. Evaluation at these higher levels of the affective domain is more difficult, for it requires observation of student behavior over time to determine if there is commitment to act according to a value system compatible with the practice of nursing. Test items are not appropriate for these levels, as the teacher is concerned with the *use* of values and motivation to carry out behaviors consistent with them.

A description and sample objective for each of the five levels of learning in the affective taxonomy follow. While sublevels have been established for each of these levels, only the five major categories are essential to guide the teacher for instructional and evaluation purposes.

1. *Receiving*: Awareness of values, attitudes, and beliefs important in nursing practice. Sensitivity to a client, clinical situation, or problem.
   The student expresses an awareness of the need for maintaining confidentiality of patient information.

2. *Responding*: Reacting to a situation. Responding voluntarily to a given phenomenon reflecting a choice made by the learner.
   The student shares willingly feelings about caring for a dying patient.

3. *Valuing*: Internalization of a value. Acceptance of a value and commitment to using it as a basis for behavior.
   The learner supports the rights of clients to their own lifestyles and decisions about care.

4. *Organization*: Development of a complex system of values. Organization of a value system.
   The learner forms a position about issues surrounding cost and quality of care.

5. *Characterization by a value*: Internalization of a value system providing a philosophy for practice.
   The learner acts consistently to involve clients and families in decision making about care.

Psychomotor Domain

Psychomotor learning involves the development of skills and competency in use of technology. This domain includes activities that are movement-oriented, requiring some degree of physical coordination. Motor skills have a cognitive base, the principles underlying the performance of the skill, and an affective dimension, reflecting the values and attitudes of the nurse while carrying out the skill, for instance, concern and respect for the client during performance of the skill (Oermann, 1991).

Different taxonomies have been developed for evaluation of psychomotor skills. An early one by Simpson (1966) included five stages in development of psychomotor skill: perception, set, guided response, mechanism, and complex overt response. Other psychomotor taxonomies have been proposed by Harrow (1972) and Kibler, Barker, and Miles (1970). A useful taxonomy for nursing was developed by Dave (1970). This taxonomy specifies five broad levels in the progression of psychomotor competency: imitation, manipulation, precision, articulation, and naturalization. A description of each of these levels and sample objectives follow.

1. *Imitation*: Performance of skill following demonstration by teacher or through multimedia. Imitative learning.
   The student follows the example for changing the dressing.
2. *Manipulation*: Ability to follow instructions rather than needing to observe the procedure or skill.
   The student suctions a patient according to accepted procedure.
3. *Precision*: Ability to perform skill accurately, independently, and without using a model or set of directions.
   The student takes vital signs accurately.
4. *Articulation*: Coordinated performance of skill within a reasonable time frame.
   The learner demonstrates skill in suctioning patients with varying health problems.
5. *Naturalization*: High degree of proficiency. Integration of skill within care.
   The learner carries out competently skills needed for care of technology-dependent children in their homes.

Evaluation methods for psychomotor skills provide data on student understanding of the cognitive base of the skill and their ability to carry out the procedure in simulated settings and with clients. The majority of these evaluation strategies are categorized as clinical evaluation methods. Test questions, however, may be used for evaluating principles associated with performing the skill—the related cognitive base.

USE OF OBJECTIVES FOR EVALUATION
AND TESTING

As described earlier, these taxonomies provide a framework for the teacher to plan instruction and design evaluation at different levels of learning, from simple to complex in the cognitive domain; from awareness of a value to developing a philosophy of practice based on internalization of a value system in the affective domain; and increasing competency, from imitation of the skill to performance as a natural part of care, in the psychomotor domain. These taxonomies are of value in designing the evaluation protocol to gear tests and other evaluation methods to the level of learning anticipated from the instruction. If the outcome of learning is application, then test items also need to be at the application level. If the outcome of learning is valuing, then the evaluation methods need to examine students' behaviors over a period of time to determine if they are committed to practice reflecting professional values and if they act on them consistently. If the outcome of skill learning is precision, then evaluation strategies need to focus on accuracy in performance, not the speed with which the skill is performed. The taxonomies, therefore, provide a useful framework to assure that test items and evaluation methods are at the appropriate level for the intended learning outcomes.

In developing test questions and other types of evaluation methods, the teacher identifies first the objective to be evaluated, then designs test items, or other evaluation strategies as appropriate, to measure that objective. The objective specifies the behavior, at a particular taxonomic level, to be evaluated and the content area to which it relates. Ebel and Frisbie (1991) defined this as objective-referenced testing. For the objective *Identifies characteristics of premature ventricular contractions,* the test item would examine student ability to recall these characteristics. The behavior "identifies" at the knowledge level indicates that recall of facts is needed to answer the question, and not comprehension nor use of this knowledge in new client situations. The content area, "characteristics of premature ventricular contractions," indicates the content to be tested.

Some teachers choose not to use the objectives as the basis for testing and evaluation and instead develop test questions and other evaluation methods from the content of the course. With this process the teacher identifies explicit content areas to be evaluated; test items then sample student knowledge of this content. Ebel and Frisbie (1991) cautioned faculty that use of content areas for this purpose requires explicit identification of the content to be tested. After identifying the content, the teacher can refer to the objectives for decisions about the level of complexity of the test questions and other methods of evaluation.

Throughout this book, multiple types of test questions and other evaluation strategies are presented. It is assumed that these items were developed from specific instructional objectives or explicit content areas. Regardless of whether the teacher uses objectives or content domains as the framework for testing and evaluation, test items and other strategies should evaluate the learning outcome intended from the instruction. This outcome specifies a behavior to be evaluated, at a particular level of complexity indicated by the taxonomic level, and a content area to which it relates. The behavior and content area provide the framework for developing test items and other evaluation methods.

SUMMARY

Evaluation is an integral part of the educational process in nursing. Through evaluation and measurement, the teacher makes important decisions about learners. Evaluation is the process of making value judgments about learners; value, in fact, is part of the word *evaluation*. Evaluation fulfills two major roles in the classroom and clinical setting: formative and summative. A third role of evaluation, confirmative, reflects continuing evaluation of learners to determine if they have maintained their clinical skills.

Measurement is the process of assigning numbers to represent student achievement according to certain rules. It answers the question, "How much?" There are two main ways of interpreting test scores and other types of evaluation conducted in the clinical setting, norm- and criterion-referenced. In norm-referenced measurement, test scores and other evaluation data are referenced to a norm group. The scores are interpreted by comparing them to those of other individuals. Norm-referenced clinical evaluation compares students' clinical performance with that of a group of learners, indicating that learners have more or less clinical competence than others in their group. Criterion-referenced measurement, on the other hand, involves interpreting scores based on preset criteria, not in relation to a group of learners. With this type of measurement, an individual score is compared to a preset standard or criterion. With criterion-referenced clinical evaluation, student performance is compared with a set of criteria to be met. Tests are one form of measurement. A test is a set of items each with a correct answer.

Instructional objectives play an important role in teaching and evaluating students in varied settings in nursing. They provide guidelines for student learning and instruction and the basis for evaluating learning. The objectives represent the outcomes of learning; these outcomes may include the acquisition of knowledge, development of values, and performance of psychomotor and technological skills. Evaluation serves to determine the extent of the student's learning in relation to these outcomes. Each of the domains of learning, cognitive, affective, and psychomotor, has its own classification or taxonomic system. The taxonomies are of value in designing test items and other evaluation strategies to gear testing and evaluation to the level of learning anticipated from the instruction. While different methods have been proposed for developing test items and other evaluation strategies, the important principle is that they relate to the learning outcomes.

REFERENCES

Bevil, C. A. (1991). Program evaluation in nursing education: Creating a meaningful plan. In M. Garbin (Ed.), *Assessing educational outcomes* (pp. 53–67). New York: National League for Nursing.

Bloom, B. S., Englehart, M. D., Furst, E. J., Hill, W. H., & Krathwohl, D. R. (1956). *Taxonomy of educational objectives: The classification of educational goals: Handbook I. Cognitive domain*. New York: David McKay.

Bott, P. A. (1996). *Testing and assessment in occupational and technical education*. Boston: Allyn and Bacon.

Dave, R. H. (1970). Psychomotor levels. In R. J. Armstrong (Ed.), *Developing and writing behavioral objectives*. Tucson, AZ: Educational Innovators Press.

Ebel, R. L. (1965). *Measuring educational achievement*. Englewood Cliffs, NJ: Prentice Hall.

Ebel, R. L., & Frisbie, D. A. (1991). *Essentials of educational measurement* (5th ed.). Englewood Cliffs, NJ: Prentice Hall.

Gronlund, N. E., & Linn, R. L. (1990). *Measurement and evaluation in teaching* (6th ed.). New York: Macmillan.

Harrow, A. J. (1972). *A taxonomy of the psychomotor domain: A guide for developing behavioral objectives*. New York: McKay.

Hellebrandt, J., & Russell, J. D. (1993). Confirmative evaluation of instructional materials and learners. *Performance & Instruction, 32* (6), 22–27.

Keith, N. Z. (1991). Assessing educational goals: The national movement to outcomes evaluation. In M. Garbin (Ed.), *Assessing educational outcomes* (pp. 1–23). New York: National League for Nursing.

Kibler, R. J., Barker, L. L., & Miles, D. T. (1970). *Behavioral objectives and instruction*. Boston: Allyn & Bacon.

Krathwohl, D., Bloom, B., & Masia, B. (1964). *Taxonomy of educational objectives: The classific of educational goals: Handbook II: Affective domain*. New York: David McKay.

Kubiszyn, T., & Borich, G. (1993). *Educational testing and measurement* (4th ed.). New York: HarperCollins.

Mitchell, R. (1992). *Testing for learning*. New York: Free Press.

Oermann, M. H. (1991). Psychomotor skill development. *Journal of Continuing Education in Nursing, 21,* 202–204.

Orchard, C. (1994). The nurse educator and the nursing student: A review of the issue of clinical evaluation procedures. *Journal of Nursing Education, 33,* 245–251.

Reilly, D. E., & Oermann, M. H. (1990). *Behavioral objectives: Evaluation in nursing* (3rd ed.). New York: National League for Nursing.

Reilly, D. E., & Oermann, M. H. (1992). *Clinical teaching in nursing education* (2nd ed.). New York: National League for Nursing.

Simpson, E. J. (1966). The classification of educational objectives: Psychomotor domain. *Illinois Teacher of Home Economics, 10,* 135–140.

Tanner, C. A. (1994). Professional judgment in evaluation. *Journal of Nursing Education, 33,* 243.

2

Qualities of Effective Measurement Instruments

How does a teacher know if a test or other measurement instrument is "good"? If the results of measurement procedures will be used to make important educational decisions, teachers must have confidence in their interpretations of test scores. Good measurement tools produce results that are valid and reliable, concepts that are important to the interpretation of measurement outcomes. In addition, measurement tools should be practical and easy to use. This chapter explains the concepts of validity and reliability and their effects on the interpretive quality of measurement results. It also discusses important practical considerations that might affect the choice or development of tests and other instruments.

VALIDITY

An understanding of the concept of validity is critical to the fair and proper use of tests (Ebel & Frisbie, 1991). Tests and other measurement instruments yield scores that teachers use to make inferences about how much the test-takers know or what they can do. Validity refers to the extent to which these score-based inferences are sound. In other words, test scores are valid if they permit the teacher to make accurate interpretations about a test-taker's knowledge or ability. Validity is not a static property of the test itself, but rather, it refers to the ways in which teachers interpret and use the test results (Nitko, 1996).

Validity is not an either/or judgment; there are degrees of validity depending on the purpose of the test and how the scores are to be used. A single test may be used for many different purposes, and the resulting test scores may have greater validity for one purpose than for another (Nitko, 1996). For example, a test designed to measure knowledge of perioperative nursing standards may produce scores that have validity for the purpose of determining certification for perioperative staff nurses, but it may yield scores that are less valid for assigning grades to students in a perioperative nursing elective course.

In order to make good judgments about the valid use of a set of scores, teachers must gather one or more types of validity evidence, a process known as validation (Ebel & Frisbie, 1991). Although a variety of evidence might be available, most could be categorized into one of these types: content-related, criterion-related, and construct-related. Each type of evidence will be discussed separately; however, they are related concepts. It is important to remember that the evidence itself does not constitute validity. Rather, validity is "a judgment you make after considering evidence from all relevant sources" (Nitko, 1996, p. 37). In addition, the validity evidence may change over time, so that validation of test scores must not be considered a one-time event.

Content-Related Evidence

Content-related evidence demonstrates the degree to which the sample of test items or tasks represents the domain of content or abilities that the teacher wants to measure (American Psychological Association [APA], 1985; Ebel & Frisbie, 1991). The term "content-related" also will be used here to apply to instruments designed to measure attitudes and psychomotor skills.

Tests and other measurement instruments usually contain only a sample of all possible items that could be used to measure the domain of interest. However, interpretations of test scores are based on what the teacher believes is the universe of items that could have been generated. In other words, when a student correctly answers 83% of items on a maternity nursing final examination, the teacher usually infers that the student would probably correctly answer 83% of all items in the universe of maternity nursing content.

A superficial conclusion could be made about the match between a test's appearance and its intended use by asking a panel of experts to judge whether the test appears to be based on appropriate content. This type of judgment, sometimes referred to as "face validity," is not sufficient evidence of content representativeness. Content-related evidence of validity should be obtained through (a) a series of test-development procedures designed to assure content representativeness and (b) *post facto* appraisals of the resulting content (Popham, 1990).

Efforts to include suitable content on the test can be made during test development. This process begins with defining the universe of content. The content definition should be related to the purpose for which the test will be used. For example, if a test is supposed to measure a new staff nurse's understanding of hospital safety policies and procedures presented during orientation, then the teacher first defines the universe of content by outlining the knowledge about policies that the staff nurse needs in order to function satisfactorily. The teacher then uses professional judgment to write or select test items that satisfactorily represent this desired content domain. A system for documenting this process, the construction of a test blueprint or table of specifications, is described in chapter 3.

After the test is constructed, judgments about the representativeness of its content can be made by asking a panel of experts to review the test, item by item, to see if the items satisfactorily represent the domain as it was defined. Both the specifications for development and the test items themselves are necessary for this validation process (Ebel & Frisbie, 1991; Popham, 1990).

Content-related evidence is necessary but not sufficient for validation. Factors other than the representativeness and relevance of the test items can influence test scores. The testing environment or student characteristics may affect the scores. For example, students with high levels of test anxiety or limited English skills may achieve scores that do not accurately represent their levels of knowledge. A noisy test environment may be distracting to students with certain learning disabilities and may need to be considered as an alternative explanation for their low scores. Although the most plausible explanation for low test scores may be insufficient knowledge of the content domain, the teacher must be able to show that these other factors do not influence the scores excessively (Ebel & Frisbie, 1991).

Criterion-Related Evidence

Criterion-related evidence illustrates that scores on the test of interest are systematically related to one or more criterion measures or outcome criteria (APA, 1985). Criterion-related validity evidence is based on the extent to which students' test scores allow the teacher to infer their performance on an independent criterion variable. For example, graduate program admissions committees often use scores from an aptitude test such as the Graduate Record Examination or Miller Analogies Test to predict whether applicants are likely to be successful in graduate school (the criterion measure).

There are two forms of criterion-related evidence: concurrent and predictive. Concurrent evidence determines the student's present standing on a criterion measure, and predictive evidence gauges the student's probable future performance on an outcome criterion. Thus the difference between the two forms concerns the time period during which the criterion data are collected. The type of evidence needed for a given test depends on how the test scores will be used. The example given above related to testing applicants to a graduate program calls for predictive validity evidence. In nursing education programs, teachers typically want to make such predictions of future performance. On the other hand, concurrent validity evidence may be desirable for making a decision about whether one test or measurement instrument may be substituted for another. For example, a staff development educator may want to collect concurrent validity evidence to determine if a checklist with a rating scale can be substituted for a less efficient narrative appraisal instrument to measure a staff nurse's job performance.

To be considered adequate, criterion measures must have certain characteristics. They must be relevant; that is, they must reflect important aspects of the variable of interest. In some cases, adequate criterion measures are not available; the test in use is considered to be the best instrument that has been devised to measure the ability in question. If better measures were available, they might be used instead of the test being validated. In other cases, appropriate criteria may be difficult to define and to measure impartially (Ebel & Frisbie, 1991). For example, a written test cannot measure many of the characteristics thought to be important to good nursing practice, but it might be difficult, if not impossible, to get a group of nurse educators to agree on an acceptable criterion measure for good nursing care—let alone to judge this ability in the same way.

Criterion measures must also be reliable; that is, they must measure the variable of interest consistently. Thus, validity evidence includes information about how reliably the criterion measure performs. The next major section of this chapter discusses the concept of reliability in more detail.

The relationship between test scores and those obtained on the criterion measure is usually expressed as a correlation coefficient. A desired level of correlation between the two measures cannot be recommended, because the correlation may be influenced by a number of factors, including test length. The teacher who uses the test must use good professional judgment to determine what magnitude of correlation is considered adequate for the intended use of the test being validated.

In any case, criterion-related evidence cannot take the place of content-related evidence. Content-related evidence should be used as primary support for the validity of test scores, but correlation with criterion measures may be useful in providing secondary, confirming evidence. After all, what a test measures is determined chiefly by the tasks included in it.

Construct-Related Evidence

Construct-related evidence refers to the extent to which the test being validated measures the construct of interest (APA, 1985). A construct is a theoretical conceptualization about an aspect of human behavior that cannot be measured directly (Ebel & Frisbie, 1991). Many variables of interest to teachers are constructs, such as critical thinking, creativity, and test anxiety. Construct-related validity evidence supports the contention that the test scores actually mean what they are intended to mean.

For example, if the purpose of a test is to measure students' ability to think critically about pediatric clinical problems, the validity evidence must show that the test items require students to demonstrate critical thinking ability. Students who achieve high scores on this test would be assumed to be better critical thinkers than students who achieve low scores. To collect evidence in support of this assumption, the teacher might design a study to predict that if the test does what it is supposed to do, students should obtain scores on the test based on their observed critical thinking behavior in clinical practice. Popham (1990) described this approach as a differential-population study. The teacher could divide the sample of students into two groups based on their clinical evaluation ratings: those who were rated by their clinical instructors as good critical thinkers in clinical practice, and those who were rated as weak critical thinkers. Then the teacher would compare the test scores of the students in both groups. If the teacher's hypothesis is confirmed, that is, if students with good clinical ratings obtain high test scores, this evidence can be used to support the validity of using the test scores to make inferences about students' critical thinking abilities.

Construct-related evidence should not be obtained through a single study of this type. Because constructs are covert, unobservable attributes, decisions about construct-related validity should be based on an accumulation of data over a period of time.

RELIABILITY

"Reliability" refers to the consistency of test scores, the extent to which they are accurate, error-free, and stable. Reliable test scores are reproducible and generalizable to other testing occasions. If a test produces reliable scores, the same group of students would achieve approximately the same scores if the test was given on another occasion. A reliability coefficient can be used to express the correlation between the two sets of scores (Ebel & Frisbie, 1991).

As the previous section of the chapter indicated, reliability is an important aspect of validity. In order for test scores to allow valid inferences, they must be reliable. So reliability is a necessary condition for validity. Reliability is not, however, a sufficient condition for validity. An example may help to illustrate the relationship between these two concepts.

Suppose that the author of this chapter was given a test of her knowledge of measurement principles. The author of a textbook on measurement and evaluation in nursing education might be expected to achieve a high score on such a test, if there is sufficient content-related evidence of validity. However, if the test was written in the Chinese language, the author's score might be very low, even if she was a remarkably good guesser, because she cannot read Chinese. If the same test was administered the following week, and every week for a month, her scores would likely be consistently low. Therefore, these test scores would be considered reliable, because there would be a high correlation among scores obtained on the same test over a period of several administrations. But a valid score-based interpretation of the author's knowledge of measurement principles could not be drawn, because the test was not appropriate for its intended use.

Test scores may be inconsistent because the behavior being measured is unstable, because the sample of test items varies, or because the scoring procedures are inconsistent. Therefore, when teachers interpret test scores, they need to have some understanding of the factors that may cause their inconsistency.

For purposes of understanding sources of inconsistency, it is helpful to view a test score as having two components, a true score and an error score, represented by the following equation:

$$X = T + E \qquad \text{[Equation 2.1]}$$

A student's actual test score (X) is also known as the observed score. That student's hypothetical true score (T) cannot be measured directly, because it is the average of all scores the student would obtain if tested on many occasions with the same test. The observed score contains a certain amount of measurement error (E), which also cannot be measured directly. Measurement error, therefore, is the difference between the observed score and the hypothetical true score (Gaberson, 1996). The amount of measurement error can be estimated from the score variance, that is, the square of the standard deviation of a set of scores (a measure of score variability). If there is little measurement error in a set of scores, differences between individual students' scores can be attributed to differences in knowledge or ability as measured by the test. If the measurement error is large, however, score differences might be attributed to random errors that are unrelated to the students' knowledge or ability (Ebel & Frisbie, 1991).

For example, Matt obtains a higher score than Kelly on a community health nursing unit test because Matt truly knows more about the content than Kelly does. Test scores should reflect this kind of difference, and if the difference in knowledge is the only explanation for the score difference, no error is involved. However, there may be other potential explanations for the difference in test scores. Matt may have obtained an unauthorized advance copy of the test; knowing which items would be included, he had the opportunity to focus his study on just the content that would be tested. Kelly may have worked overtime the night before the test and did not get enough sleep to allow her to feel alert during the test; her test performance was affected by her fatigue and decreased ability to concentrate. One goal of test designers is to maximize the amount of score variance that explains real differences in ability and minimize the amount of random error variance of scores.

Consistency or Stability

Most teachers think of reliability as consistency over time. That is, evidence of stability indicates whether students would achieve essentially the same scores if they took the same test at another time—a test–retest procedure. The correlation between the set of scores obtained on the first administration and the set obtained on the second yields a test–retest reliability coefficient. This type of reliability evidence is known as stability, and is appropriate for situations in which the trait being measured is expected to be stable over time (Ebel & Frisbie, 1991). In nursing education settings, the test-retest method of obtaining reliability information may have limited usefulness. If the same test items are used on both tests, students' answers on the retest are not independent of their answers on the first test. That is, their responses to the second test may be influenced to some extent by recall of their previous responses, or by discussion or individual review of content after the first test. In addition, if there is a long interval between testing occasions, other factors, such as real changes in student ability as a result of learning, may affect the retest scores.

Alternate-Form or Equivalent-Form Reliability

Another type of reliability evidence, alternate- or equivalent-form reliability, involves the use of two or more forms of the same test. Both forms
of the test are administered to the same group of students, and the resulting scores are correlated. A high reliability coefficient indicates that the two
forms sample the domain of content equally well. The major weakness of
this form of reliability estimate is that most teachers do not find time to
prepare two forms of the same test, let alone to assure that these forms are
indeed equivalent. Equivalent forms must be developed according to the
same test blueprint so that the content domain sampling is essentially the
same. Standardized tests typically do provide alternate forms so that test
security is not compromised. When alternate forms are used, teachers
assume that an individual who would take both forms of the test would
likely obtain consistent scores (Ebel & Frisbie, 1991; Popham, 1990).

Internal Consistency

Because most teachers cannot use alternate forms of the same test, another
type of reliability evidence, internal consistency, may be more useful. The
previously discussed types of estimating reliability involve two separate
tests. Internal consistency methods can be used with a set of scores from
only one administration of a single test. Sometimes referred to as split-half
methods, estimates of internal consistency reveal the extent to which the
test items are internally consistent or homogeneous.

The split-half technique consists of dividing the test into two equal subtests. This is usually done by including odd-numbered items on one subtest and even-numbered items on the other. Then the subtests are scored
separately, and the two subscores are correlated. The resulting correlation
coefficient is an estimate of the extent to which the two halves consistently
perform the same measurement. Longer tests tend to produce more reliable results than short tests, in part because they tend to sample the content domain more fully. Therefore, a split-half reliability estimate tends to
underestimate the true reliability of the scores produced by the whole test,
since each subtest includes only half of the total number of items. This
underestimate can be corrected by using the Spearman-Brown prophesy
formula (Popham, 1990, pp. 132–133), also called the Spearman-Brown
double-length formula (Nitko, 1996, pp. 68–69):

$$\frac{2 \times \text{correlation between half test scores}}{1 + \text{correlation between half test scores}} \quad \text{[Equation 2.2]}$$

Another method of estimating the internal consistency of a test is to use one of the Kuder-Richardson procedures, which represent the average correlation obtained from all possible split-half reliability estimates (Popham, 1990). The computation of Formula 20 (K-R20) involves information about the difficulty (proportion of correct responses) of each test item and therefore usually requires a computer. If the test items are not expected to vary much in difficulty, the simpler Formula 21 (K-R21) can be used to approximate the value of K-R20, although it will in most cases produce a slightly lower estimate of reliability. To use either formula, test items must be scored dichotomously, that is, right or wrong (Ebel & Frisbie, 1991; Nitko, 1996; Popham, 1990). If this condition cannot be met, coefficient alpha can be used to provide a reliability estimate for a test in which items could receive a range of points.

Scorer Reliability

Depending on the type of test or other measurement instrument used, error may arise from the procedures or persons used to score a test. Teachers may need to collect evidence to answer the question "Would this student have obtained the same score if a different person had scored the test or judged the performance?" The easiest method for collecting this evidence is to have two persons score each student's paper or rate each student's performance. The two scores are then compared to produce a percentage of agreement or correlated to produce an index of scorer consistency, depending on whether agreement in an absolute sense or a relative sense is required.

FACTORS THAT INFLUENCE RELIABILITY OF SCORES

From the previous discussion, it is obvious that various factors can influence the reliability of a set of test scores. These factors can be categorized into three main sources: test, student, and test administration conditions.

Test-related factors include the length of the test, homogeneity of test content, and difficulty and discrimination ability of the individual items. In general, the greater the number of test items, the greater the score reliability. Of course, adding test items to increase score reliability may be counterproductive after a certain point. According to Ebel and Frisbie (1991, p. 89), if a 5-item test produces a score reliability of 0.20, adding 60 items will increase the reliability estimate to 0.80. After that point, however, adding items will increase the reliability only slightly, and student fatigue and boredom may actually introduce more measurement error. Score reliability also is enhanced by homogeneity of content covered by the test. Course content that is tightly organized and highly interrelated tends to make homogeneous test content easier to achieve. Finally, the technical quality of test items, their difficulty, and their ability to discriminate between students who know the content and students who do not also affect the reliability of scores. Moderately difficult items that discriminate well between high achievers and low achievers and that contain no technical errors contribute a great deal to score reliability.

Student-related factors include the heterogeneity of the student group, testwiseness, and motivation. In general, reliability tends to increase as the range of talent in the group of students increases. Therefore, in situations where students are very similar to one another in ability, such as in graduate school, tests are likely to produce scores with somewhat lower reliability than desired. A student's test-taking skill and experience may also influence score reliability to the extent that the student is able to obtain a higher score than true ability would predict. The effect of motivation on reliability relates to the extent to which it influences individual students differently. If some students are not motivated to put forth their best efforts on an exam, their actual achievement levels may not be accurately represented, and their relative achievement in comparison to other students will be difficult to judge.

Teachers need to control test administration conditions in order to enhance the reliability of test scores. Inadequate time to complete the test can lower the reliability of scores, because some students who know the content will be unable to respond to all of the items. Cheating also contributes random errors to test scores when students are able to respond correctly to items to which they actually do not know the answer. Cheating, therefore, has the effect of raising the offenders' observed scores above their true scores, contributing to inaccurate and less meaningful interpretations of test scores (Ebel & Frisbie, 1991).

Because a reliability coefficient is an indication of the amount of measurement error associated with a set of scores, it is useful information for evaluating the meaning and usefulness of those scores. There is no absolute numerical value of a reliability coefficient that can be recommended as a cut-off for accepting this evidence; the usefulness of reliability information is a decision based on the purpose for which the test scores will be used. It is also important to remember that the numerical value of a reliability coefficient is not a stable property; it will fluctuate from one sample of students to another.

PRACTICALITY

Although reliability and validity are used to describe the ways in which scores are interpreted and used, practicality is a quality of the instrument itself and its administration procedures. Measurement procedures should be efficient and economical. A test is practical or usable to the extent that it is easy to administer and score, does not take too much time away from other instructional activities, and has reasonable resource requirements (Cangelosi, 1990).

Whether they develop their own tests and other measurement tools or use published instruments, teachers should focus on the following questions to help guide the selection of appropriate assessment procedures (Nitko, 1996; Popham, 1990):

1. *Is the test easy to construct and use?* Essay test items may be written more quickly and easily than multiple-choice items, but they will take more time to score. Multiple-choice items that assess a student's ability to think critically about clinical problems are time-consuming to construct, but they may be machine-scored quickly and accurately. The teacher must decide what is the best use of the time available for test construction, administration, and scoring. If a published test is selected for confirmatory evaluation of students' competencies just prior to graduation, is it practical to use? Does proper administration of the test require special training? Are the test administration directions easy to understand?

2. *Is the time needed to administer and score the test and interpret the results reasonable?* A teacher of a 15-week course wants to give a weekly 10-point quiz that would be reviewed immediately and self-scored by students; these procedures would take 30 minutes of class time. Is that the best use of instructional time? The teacher may decide that there is enormous value in the immediate feedback provided to students during the test review, and that the opportunity to obtain weekly information about the effectiveness of instruction is also beneficial; to that teacher, 30 minutes weekly is time well spent on evaluation. Another teacher, whose total instructional time is only 4 days, may find that administering more than one test consumes time that is needed for teaching. Evaluation is an important step in the instructional process, but it cannot replace teaching. As Nitko (1996) pointed out, "You can't fatten a calf by weighing it!" (p. 42).

3. *Are the costs associated with test construction, administration, and scoring reasonable?* While teacher-made tests may seem to be less expensive than published instruments, the cost of the instructor's time spent in test development must be taken into consideration. Additional costs associated with scoring of teacher-made tests must also be calculated. What is the initial cost of purchasing test booklets for published instruments, and can test booklets be reused? What is the cost of answer sheets, and does that cost include scoring services? Sometimes test publishers offer volume discounts that may benefit larger educational programs; reduced

prices for purchasing test materials and scoring services may also be available.

4. *Can the test results be interpreted easily and accurately by those who will use them?* If teachers score their own tests, will they obtain results that will help them to interpret the test scores accurately? In other words, will they have test statistics that will help them make meaning out of the individual test scores? Scanners and software are available that will quickly score exams that use certain types of answer sheets, but the scope of the information produced in the score report varies considerably. Purchased tests that are scored by the publisher also yield reports of test results; are these reports useful for their intended purpose? What information is needed or desired by the teachers who will make evaluation decisions, and is that information provided by the score-reporting service? Examples of information on score reports include individual raw total scores, individual raw subtest scores, group mean and median scores, individual or group profiles, and individual standard scores. Will the teachers who receive the reports need special training in order to interpret this information accurately? Some test publishers restrict the purchase of instruments to users with certain educational and experience qualifications, in part so that the test results will be interpreted and used properly.

SUMMARY

Because test results are often used to make important educational decisions, teachers must have confidence in their interpretations of test scores. Good measurement tools produce results that are valid and reliable.

Test scores are valid if they permit the teacher to make accurate interpretations about a test-taker's knowledge or ability. Validity is not a static property of the test itself, but rather, it refers to the ways in which teachers interpret and use the test results. Validity is not an either/or judgment; there are degrees of validity depending on the purpose of the test and how the scores are to be used. A single test may be used for many different purposes, and the resulting test scores may have greater validity for one purpose than for another.

In order to make good judgments about the valid use of a set of scores, teachers must gather one or more types of validity evidence: content-related, criterion-related, and construct-related. Content-related evidence demonstrates the extent to which the sample of test items or tasks represents the domain of content or abilities that the teacher wants to measure. Content-related evidence of validity may be obtained during the test-development process as well as by appraising the resulting content.

Criterion-related evidence illustrates that scores on the test of interest are related to one or more criterion measures or outcome criteria. Two forms of criterion-related evidence, concurrent and predictive, may be obtained. Concurrent evidence determines the student's present standing on a criterion measure, and predictive evidence gauges the student's probable future performance on an outcome criterion. Construct-related evidence refers to the extent to which the test being validated measures the construct of interest. A construct is a theoretical conceptualization about an attribute that cannot be measured directly, such as critical thinking or creativity. Construct-related validity evidence supports the contention that the test scores actually mean what they are intended to mean.

Reliability refers to the extent to which test scores are accurate, error-free, and stable. Reliable test scores are reproducible and generalizable to other testing occasions. If a test produces reliable scores, the same group of students would achieve approximately the same scores if the test was given again. A reliability coefficient can be used to express the correlation between the two sets of scores. The type of reliability evidence known as stability is appropriate for situations in which the trait being measured is expected to be stable over time. Evidence of stability indicates whether students would achieve essentially the same scores if they took the same test at another time. The correlation between the set of scores obtained on the first administration and the set obtained on the second yields a test-retest reliability coefficient. Another type of reliability evidence, alternate- or equivalent-form reliability, involves the use of two or more forms of the same test. Both forms are administered to the same group of students, and the resulting scores are correlated. A high reliability coefficient indicates that the two forms sample the domain of content equally well. Because most teachers do not have alternate forms of the same test, another type of reliability evidence, internal consistency, may be more useful. Internal consistency methods can be used with a set of scores from only one administration of a single test. Sometimes referred to as split-half methods, estimates of internal consistency reveal the extent to which the test items are internally consistent or homogeneous.

Various factors can influence the reliability of a set of test scores. These factors can be categorized into three main sources: test, student, and test administration conditions. Test-related factors include the length of the test, the homogeneity of test content, and the difficulty and discrimination ability of the individual items. Student-related factors include the heterogeneity of the student group, testwiseness, and motivation. Factors related to test administration include inadequate time to complete the test and cheating.

In addition, measurement tools should be practical and easy to use. While reliability and validity are used to describe the ways in which scores are interpreted and used, practicality is a quality of the instrument itself and of its administration procedures. Measurement procedures should be efficient and economical. Teachers need to evaluate the following factors: ease of construction and use; time needed to administer and score the test and interpret the results; costs associated with test construction, administration, and scoring; and the ease with which test results can be interpreted easily and accurately by those who will use them.

REFERENCES

American Psychological Association. (1985). *Standards for educational and psychological testing.* Washington, DC: Author.

Cangelosi, J. S. (1990). *Designing tests for evaluating student achievement.* New York: Longman.

Ebel, R. L., & Frisbie, D. A. (1991). *Essentials of educational measurement* (5th ed.). Englewood Cliffs, NJ: Prentice Hall.

Gaberson, K. B. (1996). Test design: Putting all the pieces together. *Nurse Educator, 21*(4), 28–33.

Nitko, A. J. (1996). *Educational assessment of students* (2nd ed.). Englewood Cliffs, NJ: Prentice Hall.

Popham, W. J. (1990). *Modern educational assessment: A practitioner's perspective* (2nd ed.). Englewood Cliffs, NJ: Prentice Hall.

3

Planning for Classroom Testing

Paul Johnson was caught by surprise when he looked at his office calendar and realized that a test for the course he was teaching was only a week away, even though he was the person who scheduled it! Thankful that he was not teaching this course for the first time, he searched his files for the test that he used last year. When he found it, a brief review showed that some of the content was outdated, and the test did not include items on the new content he had added this year. Because of a department policy that requires teachers to allow clerical staff 1 week to type a test, Paul realized that he would have to finish the necessary revisions of the test that night and submit it to be typed the next morning. Three days later when the department secretary was finished typing the test, Paul was out of town at a conference; when he returned to the office, there was no time for proofreading—the test had to be administered the next day. He begged for an exemption from the 2-day notice for photocopying, but when no one was available to do the job, Paul came in early on the morning of the test day and copied and stapled the test booklets himself.

With 5 minutes to spare, Paul rushed into the classroom and distributed the still-warm test booklets. He was still congratulating himself for meeting his deadline when the first student raised a hand with a question: "On item 1, is there a typo?" Then another student said, " I don't think that the correct answer for item 2 is there." A third student complained, "I'm missing page 2," while a fourth student stated, "There are 2 ds for item 5." Paul knew that it was going to be a long morning. But the worst was yet to come—as they were turning in their tests, students complained, "This test didn't cover the material that I thought it would cover," and "We spent a lot of class time analyzing case studies, but we were tested on memorization of facts." Paul did not look forward to the test review the following week.

Too often, teachers give little thought to the preparation of their tests until the last minute and then rush to get the job done. A test that is produced in this manner often contains items that are poorly chosen, ambiguous, and either too easy or too difficult, as well as grammatical, spelling, and other clerical errors. The solution lies in adequate planning for test construction before the item-writing phase begins, followed by careful critique of the completed test by other teachers. Table 3.1 lists the steps of the test-construction process. This chapter discusses the steps involved in planning for test construction; subsequent chapters will focus on the techniques of writing test items of various formats, assembling and administering the test, and analyzing the test results.

PURPOSE AND POPULATION

All decisions involved in planning a test are based on a teacher's knowledge of the purpose of the test and relevant characteristics of the population of learners to be tested. The purpose for the test involves why it is to be given, what it is supposed to measure, and how the test scores will be used. For example, if a test is to be used to measure the extent to which students have met learning objectives in order to determine course grades, its primary purpose is summative. If the teacher expects the course grades to reflect real differences in the amount of knowledge among students, the test must be sufficiently difficult to produce an acceptable range of scores. On the other hand, if a test is to be used primarily to provide feedback to staff nurses about their knowledge following a continuing education program, the purpose of the test is formative. Because the results will not be used to make important personnel decisions, a large range of scores is not necessary, and the test items might be of moderate or low difficulty.

A teacher's knowledge of the population that will be tested will be useful in selecting the item formats to be used, determining the length of the test and the testing time required, and selecting the appropriate scoring procedures. The term "population" is not used here in its research sense, but rather to indicate the general group of learners that will be tested. The students' reading levels, English-language literacy, visual acuity, health, and previous testing experience are examples of factors that might influence these decisions. For example, if the population to be tested is a group of five patients who have completed preoperative instruction for coronary

Table 3.1 Checklist for Test Construction

✔ Define the purpose of the test.

✔ Describe the population to be tested.

✔ Determine the optimum length of the test.

✔ Specify the difficulty and discrimination level of the test.

✔ Determine the scoring procedure or procedures to be used.

✔ Select item formats to be used.

✔ Construct a test blueprint or table of specifications.

✔ Write the test items.

✔ Have the test items critiqued.

✔ Determine the arrangement of items on the test.

✔ Write specific directions for each item format.

✔ Write general directions for the test and prepare a cover sheet.

✔ Print or type the test.

✔ Proofread the test.

✔ Reproduce the test.

✔ Prepare a scoring key.

✔ Prepare students for taking the test.

bypass graft surgery, the teacher would probably not plan to administer a test of 100 multiple-choice and matching items with a machine-scored answer sheet. However, this type of test might be most appropriate as a final course examination for a class of 75 senior nursing students.

TEST LENGTH

The length of the test is an important factor that is related to its purpose, the abilities of the students, the item formats that will be used, the amount of testing time available, and the desired reliability of the test scores. As was discussed in chapter 2, the reliability of test scores generally improves as the length of the test increases, so the teacher should attempt to include as many items as possible in order to adequately sample the content. However, if the purpose of the test is to measure knowledge of a small content domain with a limited number of objectives, fewer items will be needed to achieve an adequate sampling of content.

The test length is probably limited by the scheduled length of a testing period, so it is wise to construct the test so that the majority of students working at their normal pace will be able to attempt to answer all items (Ebel & Frisbie, 1991). This type of test is called a *power* test. A *timed* or *speeded* test is one that does not provide sufficient time for all students to respond to all items. Although most standardized tests are speeded, this type of test generally is not appropriate for teacher-made tests, in which accuracy rather than speed of response is important (Cangelosi, 1990; Ebel & Frisbie, 1991).

The item formats used and the taxonomy level that they are testing will also determine how many items should be included. Test items that require students to supply an answer, such as essay and completion items, generally require more testing time than items that require students to select an answer, such as multiple-choice and matching. Multiple-choice items with 5 options will require more reading and thinking time than items with 3 options.

DIFFICULTY AND DISCRIMINATION LEVEL

The desired difficulty of the test and its ability to differentiate among various levels of performance are related considerations. Both factors are affected by the purpose of the test and the way in which the scores will be interpreted and used. If the test results are to be interpreted in a criterion-referenced manner, the test is likely to be easier than one designed to yield norm-referenced interpretations. When testing for minimum competency, the expectation is that most students will achieve this level of performance. The test items, therefore, should be easy for the students who have mastered the content, but difficult for those who have not. The resulting distribution of test scores is likely to be homogeneous, and the ability of such a test to discriminate among various levels of performance is therefore weak (Ebel & Frisbie, 1991).

On the other hand, tests designed for norm-referenced interpretation should produce a range of scores that is more heterogeneous, revealing different levels of achievement among the students tested. Test items for this type of test, therefore, should be moderately difficult. "The ideal difficulty of these items should be at a point on the difficulty scale (percent correct) midway between perfect (100% correct response) and the chance level difficulty (50% correct for true-false items, 25% correct for four-alternative multiple-choice items)" (Ebel & Frisbie, 1991, p. 130). In other words, the moderately difficult true-false item should be answered correctly by about 75% of students.

It is important to keep in mind that the difficulty level of test items can only be estimated in advance, depending on the teacher's experience in testing this content and knowledge of the abilities of the students to be tested. Procedures for determining how the test items actually perform are discussed in chapter 9.

ITEM FORMATS

Some students may be particularly adept at answering essay items; others may prefer multiple-choice items. However, tests should be designed to provide information about students' knowledge or abilities, not about their skill in taking certain types of tests. A test with a variety of item formats usually provides students with more opportunity to demonstrate their achievement of the test's objectives than does a test with only a one-item format (Cangelosi, 1990, pp. 52-53). All item formats have their advantages and limitations, which are discussed in chapters 4, 5, and 6.

Most teachers tend to write test items in a format that seems most useful to them or that they feel most comfortable using (Ebel & Frisbie, 1991). Many nursing faculty members use only multiple-choice items because of a rather powerful and persistent myth: that since the licensure examination contains only multiple-choice items, nursing students must be tested exclusively with this type of item. However, although students need ample practice with multiple-choice items so that they are comfortable with this type of test prior to taking the licensure examination, multiple-choice items are not appropriate for testing all instructional objectives on teacher-made tests. Teachers should select item formats for their tests based on a variety of factors, such as the objectives to be evaluated, the specific skill to be measured, and the ability level of the students.

Some objectives are better measured with certain item formats. For example, if the instructional objective specifies that the student will be able to "Discuss the comparative advantages and disadvantages of breast- and bottle-feeding," a multiple-choice item would be inappropriate, because it would not allow the teacher to evaluate the student's ability to organize and express ideas on this topic. An essay item would be a better choice for this purpose.

The teacher's time constraints may affect the choice of item format. In general, essay items take less time to write than multiple-choice items, but they are more difficult and time-consuming to score. A teacher who has little time to prepare a test and therefore chooses an essay format, assuming that this choice is also appropriate for the objectives to be tested, must plan for considerable time after the test is given to score it.

SCORING PROCEDURES

Decisions about what scoring procedure or procedures to use are somewhat dependent on the choice of item formats. Student responses to short-answer, numerical calculation, and essay items, for instance, must be hand-scored, whether they are recorded directly on the test itself or on a separate answer sheet or booklet. Answers to objective test items such as multiple-choice, true-false, and matching also may be recorded on the test itself or on a separate answer sheet. Scannable answer sheets increase greatly the speed with which objective tests may be scored and have the additional advantage of allowing the production of computer-generated item analysis reports. The teacher should decide if the time and resources available for scoring a test suggest that hand-scoring or machine-scoring would be preferable. In any case, this decision alone should not influence the choice of test item format.

TEST BLUEPRINT

Most people would not think of building a house without blueprints. In fact, the word "house" denotes diverse attributes to different individuals. For this reason, a potential homeowner would not purchase a lot, call a builder, and say only "Build a house for me on my lot." The builder might think that a proper house consists of a 2-story brick Colonial with 4 bedrooms, 3 baths, and a formal dining room, while the homeowner had in mind a 3-bedroom ranch with 2 baths, an eat-in kitchen, and a fireplace. Similarly, the word "test" might mean different things to different teachers; students and their teacher might have widely varied expectations about what the test will contain. The best way to avoid misunderstanding regarding the nature of a test and also to ensure that highly valid scores will be obtained is to develop a test blueprint, also known as a test plan or a table of specifications, before building the test itself.

The elements of a test blueprint include (a) a list of the major topics or instructional objectives that the test will cover; (b) the level of complexity of the task to be assessed; and (c) the emphasis each topic will have, indicated by number or percentage of items or points. Figure 3.1 is an example of a test blueprint for a unit test on nursing care during normal pregnancy that illustrates each of these elements.

The row headings along the left margin of the example are the content areas that will be tested. In this case, the content is indicated by a general outline of topics. Teachers may find that a more detailed outline of content or a list of the relevant objectives is more useful for a given purpose and

CONTENT	LEVEL OF COGNITIVE SKILL[a]				
	K	C	Ap	An	Total#[b]
I. Conception and fetal development	3	2	3		8
II. Maternal physiological changes in pregnancy	2	3	1	2	8
III. Maternal psychological changes in pregnancy	3	2	2		7
IV. Social, cultural, and economic factors affecting pregnancy outcome	2	3		3	8
V. Signs and symptoms of pregnancy	2	2	2		6
VI. Antepartal nursing care	6	8	10	6	30
VII. Preparation for childbirth	3	4	1		8
TOTAL # [b]	21	24	19	11	75

Figure 3.1 Example of a test blueprint for a unit test on normal pregnancy (75 points).

[a] According to Bloom et al. (1956) taxonomy of cognitive objectives. Selected levels are included in this test blueprint and are represented by the following key:

    K = Knowledge

    C = Comprehension

    Ap = Application

    An = Analysis

[b] Number of points. Test blueprints also may include the number or the percentage of items.

population. Some teachers combine a content outline and a list of objectives; in this case, an additional column of objectives would be inserted before or after the content list.

The column headings across the top of the example are taken from a taxonomy of cognitive objectives (Bloom, Englehart, Furst, Hill, & Krathwohl, 1956). Since the test blueprint is a tool to be used by the teacher, it can be modified in any way that makes sense to the user. Accordingly, the teacher who prepared this blueprint chose to use only selected levels of the taxonomy. Other teachers might include all levels or different levels of Bloom's taxonomy, or use a different taxonomy.

The body of the test blueprint is a grid formed by the intersections of content topics and cognitive levels. Each of the cells of the grid has the potential for representing one or more test items that might be developed. The numbers in the cells of the sample test blueprint represent the number of points on the test that will relate to it; some teachers prefer to indicate numbers of items or the percentage of points or items represented by each cell. It is not necessary to write test items for each cell; the teacher's judgment concerning the appropriate emphasis and balance of content governs the decision about which cells should be filled and how many items should be written for each. Rigorous classification of items into these cells also is unnecessary and in fact, impossible (Nitko, 1996). The way in which the content is taught may affect whether the related test items will be written at the application or comprehension level. Minor adjustments in classification of items may be made after the content is taught, as long as the overall emphasis and balance of the test is preserved.

Once developed, the test blueprint serves several important functions. First, it is a useful tool for guiding the work of the item writer so that sufficient items are developed at the appropriate level to test important content areas and objectives. Using such a tool helps teachers to be accountable for the educational outcomes they produce. The test blueprint also can be used as evidence for judging the validity of the resulting test scores (Ebel & Frisbie, 1991). The completed test and blueprint may be reviewed by content experts who can judge whether the test items adequately represent the specified content domain, as described in the procedures for collecting content-related evidence in chapter 2.

Another important use of the test blueprint is to inform students about the nature of the test and how they should prepare for it. Although the content covered in class and assigned readings should give students a general idea of the content areas to be tested, students often lack a clear sense of the cognitive levels at which they will be tested on this material. While it might be argued that the instructional objectives might give students a clue as to the level at which they will be tested, teachers often forget that students are not as sophisticated in interpreting objectives as are teachers. Also, some teachers are good at writing objectives that specify a reasonable expectation of performance, but their test items may in fact test higher or lower performance levels. Students need to know the level at which they will be tested because that knowledge will affect how they prepare for the test, not necessarily how much they prepare. They should prepare differently for items that test their ability to apply information than for items that test their ability to synthesize information.

Some teachers worry that if the test blueprint is shared with students, they will not study the content areas that would contribute less to their overall test scores, preferring to concentrate their time and energy on the more important areas of emphasis. If this indeed is the outcome, is it necessarily harmful? Absent any guidance from the teacher, students unwisely may spend equal amounts of time reviewing all content areas. In fact, professional experience reveals that some knowledge is more important for use in practice than is other knowledge. Even if they are good critical thinkers, students may be unable to discriminate more important content from that which is less important because they lack the practice experience to make this distinction. Withholding information about the content emphasis of the test from students might be perceived as an attempt to threaten or punish them for perceived shortcomings such as failure to attend class, failure to read what was assigned, or failure to discern the teacher's priorities. Such a use of testing would be considered unethical.

The best time to share the test blueprint with students is at the beginning of the course or unit of study. If students are unfamiliar with the use of a test blueprint, the teacher may need to explain the concept as well as to discuss how it might be useful to the students in planning their preparation for the test. Of course, if the teacher subsequently makes modifications in the blueprint after writing the test items, those changes also should be shared with the students (Nitko, 1996).

WRITING THE TEST ITEMS

After developing the test blueprint, the teacher begins to write the test items that correspond to each cell. Regardless of the selected item formats, the teacher should consider some general factors that contribute to the quality of test items.

General Rules for Writing Test Items

1. *Every item should measure something important.* If a test blueprint is designed and used as described in the previous section, each test item will measure an important objective or content area. Without using a blueprint, teachers often write test items that test trivial or obscure knowledge. Sometimes the teacher's intent is to determine if students have read assigned materials; however, if the content is not important information, it wastes the teacher's time to write the item, and wastes the student's time to read it and respond to it. Similarly, it is not necessary to write "filler" items to meet a targeted number; a test with 98 well-written items that measure important objectives will work as well as or better than one with 98 good items and 2 meaningless ones. In fact, students who know the content well might regard a test item that measures trivial knowledge with annoyance or even suspicion, believing that it is meant to trick them into answering incorrectly.

2. *Every item should have a correct answer.* This may seem obvious, but this rule is violated frequently because of the teacher's failure to make a

distinction between fact and belief. In some cases, the correct or best answer to a test item might be a matter of opinion, and unless a particular authority is cited in the item, students might justifiably argue a different response than the one the teacher expected.

For example, one answer to the question, "When does life begin?" might be "When the kids leave home and the dog dies." If the intent of the question was to measure understanding of when a fetus becomes viable, this is not the correct answer, although if that was the teacher's intent, the question is poorly worded. There are a variety of opinions and beliefs about the concept of viability; a better way to word the question is, "According to American College of Obstetricians and Gynecologists standards, at what gestational age does a fetus become viable?" If a test item asks the student to state an opinion about an issue and to support that position with evidence, that is a different matter. The item will not be scored as correct or incorrect, but with variable credit based on the completeness of the response, rationale given for the position taken, or the soundness of the student's reasoning.

3. *Use clear, concise, precise, grammatically correct language.* Students who read the test item need to know exactly what task is required of them. Wording a test item clearly is often difficult due to the inherent abstractness and imprecision of language (Ebel & Frisbie, 1991, p. 139). The teacher should include enough detail in the test item to communicate the intent of the item, but without using extraneous words that only serve to increase reading time. Grammatical errors may provide unintentional clues to the correct response for the test-wise but unprepared student and, at best, annoy the well-prepared student.

4. *Avoid using jargon, slang, or unnecessary abbreviations.* Health care professionals frequently use jargon and abbreviations in their practice environment; in some ways it allows them to communicate more quickly, if not more effectively, with others who understand the same language. Informal language in a test item, however, may fail to communicate the intent of the item accurately. Because most students are somewhat anxious when taking tests, they may fail to interpret an abbreviation correctly for the context in which it is used.

For example, does MI mean myocardial infarction, mitral insufficiency, or Michigan? Of course, if the intent of the test item is to measure students' ability to define commonly used abbreviations, it would be appropriate to use the abbreviation in the item and ask for the definition, or give the definition and ask the student to supply the abbreviation. Slang almost always conveys the impression that the item-writer does not take the job seriously.

5. *Try to use positive wording.* It is difficult to explain this rule without using negative wording, but in general, avoid including words like "no," "not," and "except" in the test item. The use of negative wording is espe-

cially confusing in true-false items. If using a negative form is unavoidable, underline the negative word or phrase, or use bold text and all uppercase letters to draw the student's attention to it. It is best to avoid asking students to identify the incorrect response, as in the following example:

> Which of the following is NOT an indication that a skin lesion is a Stage IV pressure ulcer?
>
> a. Blistering*
> b. Sinus tracts
> c. Tissue necrosis
> d. Undermining

The structure of this item reinforces the wrong answer and may lead to confusion when a student attempts to recall the correct information at a later time. A better way to word the item is:

> Which of the following is an indication that a skin lesion is a Stage II pressure ulcer?
>
> a. Blistering*
> b. Sinus tracts
> c. Tissue necrosis
> d. Undermining

6. *No item should contain irrelevant clues to the correct answer.* This is a common error among inexperienced test item writers. Students who are good test-takers can usually identify such an item and use its flaws to improve their chances of guessing the correct answer when they do not know it. Irrelevant clues include a multiple-choice stem that is grammatically inconsistent with one or more of the options, a word in the stem that is repeated in the correct option, using qualifiers such as "always" or "never" in incorrect responses, placing the correct response in a consistent position among a set of options, or consistently making true statements longer than false statements (Nitko, 1996). Such items contribute little to the validity of test results because they may not measure what students actually know, but how well they are able to guess the correct answers.

7. *No item should depend on another item for meaning or for the correct answer.* In other words, if a student answers one item incorrectly, he or she will likely answer the related item incorrectly. An example of such a relationship between two completion items follows:

---

* Throughout this volume the asterisk indicates the correct response to the test question.

1. Which insulin should be used for emergency treatment of ketoacidosis? _____
2. What is the onset of action for the insulin in Item 1? _____

In this example, Item 2 is dependent on Item 1 for its meaning. Students who supply the wrong answer to Item 1 are unlikely to supply a correct answer to Item 2. Items should be worded in such a way as to make them independent of each other. However, a series of test items can be developed to relate to a context such as a case study, database, diagram, graph, or other interpretive material. Items that are linked to this material are called context-dependent items (Nitko, 1996, p. 138), and they do not violate this general rule for writing test items because they are linked to a common stimulus, not to each other.

8. *Arrange for critique of the items.* The best source of this critique is a colleague who teaches the same content area, or at least someone who is skilled in the technical aspects of item-writing. If no one is available to critique the test items, the teacher who developed them should set them aside for a few days. This will allow the teacher to review the items with a fresh perspective in order to identify lack of clarity or faulty technical construction.

9. *Prepare more items than the test blueprint specifies.* This will allow for replacement items for those discarded in the review process. The fortunate teacher who does not need to use many replacement items can use the remainder to begin an item bank for future tests.

PREPARING STUDENTS TO TAKE THE TEST

A teacher-made test typically measures students' maximum performance, rather than their typical performance. For this reason, teachers should create conditions under which students will be able to demonstrate their best possible performance. These conditions include adequate preparation of students to take the test (Nitko, 1996, p. 303). Although this is the last point on the test construction checklist (see Table 3.1, p. 38), the teacher should begin preparing students to take the test at the time the test is scheduled. Adequate preparation includes information, skills, and attitudes that will facilitate students' maximum performance on the test.

Students need information about the test in order to plan for effective preparation. They need sufficient time to prepare for a test, and the date and time of a test should be announced well in advance. Although many teachers believe that unannounced or "pop" tests motivate students to study more, there is no evidence to support this position. In fact, surprise tests can be considered punitive or threatening and, as such, represent an unethical use of testing (Nitko, 1996, p. 303). Adult learners with multiple responsibilities may need to make adjustments to their work and family responsibilities in order to have adequate study time, and generous notice of a planned test date will allow them to set their priorities.

In addition, students need to know about the conditions under which they are to be tested, such as how much time will be allotted, whether they will have access to resources such as textbooks, how many items will be included, the types of item formats that will be used, and if they need special tools or supplies to take the test, such as calculators, pencils, or black ink pens. Of course, students should also know what content will be covered on the test, how many items will be devoted to each content area, and the cognitive level at which they will be expected to perform. As previously discussed, giving students a copy of the test blueprint and discussing it with them is an effective way for teachers to convey this information. Students should also have sufficient opportunity to practice the type of performance that will be tested. For example, if students will be expected to solve medication dose-calculation problems without the use of a calculator, they should practice this type of calculation in class exercises or out-of-class assignments. Students also need to know if spelling, grammar, punctuation, or organization will be considered in scoring open-ended items, so that they can prepare accordingly. Finally, teachers should tell students how their test results will be used, including the weight assigned to the test score in grading (Nitko, 1996).

Another way that teachers can assist students to study for a test is to have them prepare and use a "cheat sheet." Although this term can be expected to have negative connotations for most teachers, cheat sheets are commonly used in nursing practice in the form of memory aids or triggers such as procedure checklists, pocket guides, and reminder sheets. When legitimized for use in studying and test-taking, cheat sheets capitalize on the belief that while dishonest behavior should be discouraged, the skills associated with cheating can be powerful learning tools. That is, students who plan to cheat on a test often attempt to guess potential test items and prepare crib or cheat sheets that include information to help them answer those items (de la Cruz, McKindsey, Hoffman, & Lander, 1991). Using this skill for a more honest purpose, the teacher can encourage all students to anticipate potential test items. In a test-preparation context, the teacher requires students to develop a written cheat sheet that summarizes, prioritizes, condenses, and analyzes content that they think is important and wish to remember during the test. The teacher may set parameters such as the length of the cheat sheet, for example, one side of one sheet of $8\frac{1}{2}$-by-11-inch paper. The students bring their cheat sheets on the day of the test and may use them during the test; they submit their cheat sheets along with their test papers. Students who do not submit a cheat sheet may be penalized by deducting points from the test score. Students may not even consult their cheat sheets during the test; the greatest benefit to the use of cheat sheets is in the study and preparation that goes into developing them. The teacher also may review the cheat sheets with students whose test scores are low to identify weaknesses in thinking that may have contributed to their errors; when used for this purpose, the cheat sheet becomes a powerful diagnostic and feedback tool.

With an increasingly diverse population of learners in every educational setting, including growing numbers of students for whom English is a second language and whose testing experiences may be different from the teacher's expectations, teachers should determine if students have adequate test-taking skills for the type of test to be given. If students lack adequate test-taking skill, their test scores may be lower than their actual abilities. Skill in taking tests is sometimes called testwiseness. To be more precise, testwiseness is the ability to use test-taking skills, clues from poorly written test items, and test-taking experience to achieve a test score that is higher than the student's true knowledge would predict. Common errors made by item writers do allow some students to substitute testwiseness for knowledge (Ebel & Frisbie, 1991). But, in general, all students should develop adequate test-taking skills so that they are not at a disadvantage when their scores are compared with those of more testwise individuals (Nitko, 1996).

Adequate test-taking skills include the following abilities (Ebel & Frisbie, 1991; Nitko, 1996):

1. Reading and listening to directions and following them accurately.
2. Recording answers to test items accurately and neatly.
3. Avoiding physical and mental fatigue by paced study and adequate rest before the test rather than late-night cram sessions supplemented by stimulants.
4. Using test time wisely and working at a pace that allows for careful reflection but also permits responding to all items that the student is likely to answer correctly.
5. Outlining and organizing responses to essay items before beginning to write.
6. Checking answers to test items for clerical errors and changing answers if a better response is indicated.

Many teachers advise students not to change their answers to test items, believing that the first response usually is the correct answer and that changing responses will not increase a student's score. Research findings, however, do not support this position. Studies of answer-changing and its effect on test performance (Haase, Riley, Dunn, & Gaskins, 1992; Jordan & Johnson, 1990) revealed that most students do change at least one answer on a multiple-choice test, and that more changes were made from incorrect to correct answers than from correct to incorrect. Thus, answer-changing tends to improve a student's test score. However, most students believe that changing their answers would be detrimental to their scores. Students should be encouraged to change their first response to any item when they have a good reason for making the change. For example, a student who has a clearer understanding of an item after rereading it, who later recalls additional information needed to answer the item, or who receives a clue to the correct answer from another item, should not hesitate to change the first answer (Gaskins, Dunn, Forte, Wood, & Riley, 1996; Jordan & Johnson, 1990). Improvement in test scores should not be expected when students change answers without a clear rationale for the change. Because most research studies on answer-changing related only to multiple-choice tests, further investigation of its effects on other types of tests is needed.

Finally, teachers should prepare students to approach a test with helpful attitudes. Although anxiety is a common response to situations in which performance is evaluated, high levels of anxiety are likely to interfere with maximum performance. Students need to view tests and other assessment procedures as opportunities to demonstrate what they know and what they can do. To foster this attitude, the teacher should express confidence in students' abilities to prepare for and perform well on an upcoming test. It may be helpful for the teacher to ask students what would help them to feel more relaxed and less anxious before a test. Conducting a review session and giving practice items similar to those that will be used on the test are examples of strategies that are likely to reduce students' anxiety to manageable levels (Nitko, 1996, pp. 306–307).

Whether some students can accurately be characterized as test-anxious is a controversial issue. Some teachers believe that test anxiety really is an indication of poor preparation or inadequate knowledge. However, some researchers who have studied test anxiety characterized it as a trait that has two aspects: an emotional component, or autonomic arousal, which refers to unpleasant feelings and nervousness; and the cognitive component of worry, which refers to thoughts or concerns related to expectations about performance and its consequences (Poorman & Martin, 1991). The diagnosis and treatment of test anxiety is beyond the scope of this textbook. However, teachers may be able to identify students whose performance suggests that test anxiety may be a factor, and to refer those students for treatment.

SUMMARY

Teachers who leave little time for adequate preparation often produce tests that contain poorly chosen and poorly written test items. Sufficient planning for test construction before the item-writing phase begins, followed by careful critique of the completed test by other teachers, is likely to produce a test that will yield more valid results.

All decisions involved in planning a test should be based on a teacher's knowledge of the purpose of the test and relevant characteristics of the population of learners to be tested. The purpose for the test involves why it is to be given, what it is supposed to measure, and how the test scores will be used. A teacher's knowledge of the population that will be tested will be useful in selecting the item formats to be used, determining the length of the test and the testing time required, and selecting the appropriate scoring procedures. The students' reading levels, English-language literacy, visual acuity, health, and previous testing experience are examples of factors that might influence these decisions.

The length of the test is an important factor that is related to its purpose, the abilities of the students, the item formats that will be used, the amount of testing time available, and the desired reliability of the test scores. The desired difficulty of the test and its ability to differentiate among various levels of performance are affected by the purpose of the test and the way in which the scores will be interpreted and used. If the test results are to be interpreted in a criterion-referenced manner, the test should be somewhat easier than one designed to yield norm-referenced interpretations.

A test with a variety of item formats usually provides students with more opportunity to demonstrate their achievement of the test's objectives than a test with only one item format. All item formats have advantages and limitations. Teachers should select item formats based on a variety of factors, such as the objectives, specific skill to be measured, and the ability level of the students. Some objectives are better measured with certain item formats.

Decisions about what scoring procedure or procedures to use are somewhat dependent on the choice of item formats. Student responses to some item formats must be hand-scored, whether they are recorded directly on the test itself or on a separate answer sheet or booklet. Answers to objective-type test items also may be recorded on the test itself or on a separate answer sheet. The teacher should decide if the time and resources available for scoring a test suggest that hand-scoring or machine-scoring would be preferable.

The best way to ensure that highly valid scores will be obtained is to develop a test blueprint, also known as a test plan or a table of specifications, before building the test itself. The elements of a test blueprint include (a) a list of the major topics or instructional objectives that the test will cover; (b) the level of complexity of the task to be assessed; and (c) the emphasis each topic will have, indicated by number or percentage of items or points. Once developed, the test blueprint serves several important functions. It is a useful tool for guiding the work of the item writer so that sufficient items are developed at the appropriate level to test important content areas and objectives. It also can be used as evidence for judging the validity of the resulting test scores. It should also be used to inform students about the nature of the test and how they should prepare for it.

After developing the test blueprint, the teacher begins to write the test items that correspond to it. Regardless of the selected item formats, the teacher should follow some general rules that contribute to the development of high-quality test items.

Because teacher-made tests typically measure students' maximum performance, rather than their typical performance, teachers should create conditions under which students will be able to demonstrate their best possible performance. These conditions include adequate preparation of students to take the test. Adequate preparation includes the imparting of information, skills, and attitudes that will facilitate students' maximum performance on the test.

REFERENCES

Bloom, B. S., Englehart, M. D., Furst, E. J., Hill, W. H., & Krathwohl, D. R. (1956). *Taxonomy of educational objectives: The classification of educational goals. Handbook I: Cognitive domain*. White Plains, NY: Longman.

Cangelosi, J. S. (1990). *Designing tests for evaluating student achievement*. New York: Longman.

de la Cruz, L. A. D., McKindsey, S., Hoffman, D., & Lander, J. (1991). Cheat sheets. *Nurse Educator, 16* (1), 4, 15.

Ebel, R. L., & Frisbie, D. A. (1991). *Essentials of educational measurement* (5th ed.). Englewood Cliffs, NJ: Prentice Hall.

Gaskins, S., Dunn, L., Forte, L., Wood, F., & Riley, P. (1996). Student perceptions of changing answers on multiple-choice nursing examinations. *Journal of Nursing Education, 35,* 88–90.

Haase, P. A., Riley, C. P., Dunn., L., & Gaskins, S. (1992). A review of literature on changing answers on multiple-choice examinations. In L. R. Allen (Ed.), *Review of research in nursing education* (Vol. 5, pp. 107–121). New York: National League for Nursing.

Jordan, L., & Johnson, D. (1990). The relationship between changing answers and performance on multiple-choice nursing examinations. *Journal of Nursing Education, 29,* 337–340.

Nitko, A. J. (1996). *Educational assessment of students* (2nd ed.). Englewood Cliffs, NJ: Prentice Hall.

Poorman, S. G., & Martin, E. J. (1991). The role of nonacademic variables in passing the National Council Licensure Examination. *Journal of Professional Nursing, 7,* 25–32.

4

Objective Test Items: True–False, Matching, and Short-Answer

The decision as to the types of test items and other evaluation methods to develop depends largely on the intended learning outcomes. Once the objective or content domain to be evaluated is specified, the teacher can determine the types of test questions appropriate for measuring them. Some test items are not appropriate for certain learning outcomes or levels of complexity. True–false questions, for instance, are best suited for recall of specific information and comprehension; essay items, in contrast, provide an opportunity for students to express their own ideas, analyze different points of view, and provide a rationale for their own thinking. The learning outcomes to be evaluated, therefore, are important in deciding on the type of test question. Not all objectives nor content domains need to be evaluated through testing. In some instances, test questions may not be used, and other types of evaluation methods, such as problem-solving strategies, critical incidents, papers, projects, and rating scales, to name a few, are more appropriate.

In nursing programs faculty often develop multiple-choice questions as the predominant if not the only format of test questions. Although this provides essential practice for students in preparation for taking licensing and other certification examinations, it negates the principle of selecting the most appropriate type of test item for the outcome and content to be evaluated. In addition, it limits variety in testing and creativity in evaluating student learning. Although practice with multiple-choice questions is critical, other types of test items and evaluation strategies also are appropriate for measuring student learning in nursing.

An evaluation protocol for a course should include multiple types of test items and evaluation methods to reflect the different outcomes of learning anticipated from the course and related clinical experiences. Varying the evaluation methods also enables the teacher to be creative in how learning is judged in the course, reflects the complexity of learning that takes place, and considers individual differences among students in how they respond to testing and evaluation. The evaluation planned for a course, therefore, will more than likely include multiple evaluation methods. The role the evaluation serves, formative or summative, also influences these decisions. With formative evaluation, the teacher may develop a series of short diagnostic quizzes with limited types of test questions but geared to a review of important content. In clinical practice students may complete a series of short written assignments for formative purposes. With summative evaluation, however, more extensive testing with varied types of items and other forms of evaluation may be planned to measure student achievement and certify competency in practice.

OBJECTIVE TEST ITEMS

Types of items used typically in tests may be classified as objective and essay. Objective items, which are structured and ask the student to supply an answer or choose among alternatives, include true–false, matching, short-answer, multiple-choice, and multiple-response. Essay questions provide an opportunity for students to formulate their own responses, drawing upon prior learning, and express their ideas in writing. Scoring for objective tests, however, is certainly easier and more consistent than scoring of essay and other written assignments. In addition to essay items, other types of evaluation methods appropriate for classroom use in nursing include written assignments, problem-solving strategies, critical incidents, case scenarios, and simulations. Each of these strategies will be discussed in later chapters of the book.

Although objective tests are effective for measuring knowledge of facts, understanding, application of concepts in new situations, and skill in analysis, they are not appropriate for examining ability to organize and express ideas, synthesize from varied sources, evaluate based on internal and external criteria, and develop creative solutions to problems. Objective tests require a relatively large number of items, compared with a smaller number of essay items, but provide for an extensive sampling of the content. With essay questions sampling of course content is limited because of the smaller number of test items that can be included on each examination (Gronlund & Linn, 1990, p. 124). The teacher needs to be concerned about including test items and other evaluation methods that are sufficient to adequately sample the content to be tested. Not all objectives nor content areas are tested; a test reflects instead a sampling of content. In each content area, and for each specific learning outcome, the teacher samples student performance in that area, assuming that their responses would be consistent if other items were drawn from the same content area (Gronlund & Linn, 1990, p. 129). Test items, then, should provide for an adequate sampling of each content area. In this chapter, three types of objective items are presented: true–false, matching, and short-answer. Multiple-choice and multiple-response are described in chapter 5.

TRUE–FALSE

A true–false item consists of a statement that the student judges as true or false. In some forms, students also correct a response or supply a rationale as to why the statement is true or false. True–false items are most effective for recall of facts and specific information, but also may be used to test the student's comprehension of an important principle or concept. Each item represents a declarative sentence stating a fact or principle and asking the learner to decide if it is true or false, right or wrong, or correct or incorrect. Some authors refer to this type of test item as "alternate response," allowing for these varied response formats. For affective outcomes, the agree–disagree format might be used, asking the learner to agree or disagree with a value-based statement.

There are different opinions as to the value of true–false items. Although some authors express concern over the low level of testing, focus on recall of facts, and opportunity for guessing, others indicate that true-false items provide an efficient means of examining student acquisition of knowledge in a course. Ebel and Frisbie (1991) suggest that true–false items are an effective means of testing content, as the student may answer a large number of questions in a short time. Students are able to answer between three to five true–false items per minute (Bott, 1996); as such, a large number of items may be included in a test, providing a way of testing a wide range of content. True–false items, however, are not effective discriminators between high- and low-achieving students in comparison to other types of questions such as multiple-choice (Ebel & Frisbie, 1991, p. 135).

In terms of guessing, Ebel and Frisbie (1991) differentiated blind from informed guessing, suggesting that motivated students and those who understand the content are more likely to use informed guessing. They indicated, in addition, that as the number of true–false items increases, the influence of blind guessing decreases. For instance, with one true–false item, there is a 50% chance of guessing the correct answer. As the number of items increases, however, the chance of getting a perfect score by guessing decreases to the point where on a 10-item test, it is only 0.1% (Ebel & Frisbie, 1991, p. 138).

Although true–false items are relatively easy to construct, the teacher needs to avoid using them to test meaningless information. Designed to examine student recall and comprehension of *important* facts and principles, true–false items should not be used to evaluate memorization of irrelevant information. Prior to constructing these items, the teacher might ask: Is the content evaluated by the true–false item important considering course objectives? Does the content represent knowledge taught in the class or through other methods of instruction? Is the content such that students need an understanding of it to progress through the course as a basis for further learning?

Writing True–False Items

A number of principles should be considered when writing each of the test items presented in this book. Although important principles are discussed, the lists are not intended to be inclusive; other sources on test construction might include additional helpful suggestions.

1. *The true–false item should test recall of important facts and information.* Avoid constructing items that test trivia and meaningless information. The content should be worth knowing.

2. *The statement should be true or false without qualification—*unconditionally true or false. The teacher should be able to defend the answer without conditions.

3. *Avoid words such as "usually," "sometimes," "often," and other similar ones.* Gronlund and Linn (1990) indicate that these words typically occur in true statements, giving the student clues as to the correct response. Along the same line, avoid words such as "never," "always," "all," and "none," often indicating a false response.

4. *Each item should include one idea to be tested,* rather than multiple ones. When there are different propositions to be tested, each should be designed as a single true–false item.

5. *Items should be worded precisely and clearly.* Avoid long statements with different qualifiers, and focus the sentence instead on the main idea to be tested. Long statements take time for reading and do not contribute to testing student knowledge of an important fact or principle. Develop statements that focus on the significant points to be tested.

6. *Avoid the use of negatives,* particularly double negatives. They are confusing to read and may interfere with student ability to understand the statement. For instance, the item: "It is not normal for a 2-year-old to demonstrate hand-preference" (true) would be stated more clearly as, "It is normal for a 2-year-old to demonstrate hand-preference" (false).

7. *With a series of true–false items, statements should be similar in length.* The teacher may be inclined to write longer true sentences than false ones in an attempt to state the concept clearly and precisely. Although some sources suggest including an equal number of true and false items on a test (Gronlund & Linn, 1990; Kubiszyn & Borich, 1993), others recommend including more false than true statements, considering that false statements discriminate more effectively between high- and low-achieving students (Ebel & Frisbie, 1991, p. 149; Hopkins, Stanley, & Hopkins, 1990, p. 250).

8. *Decide how to score true–false items prior to administering them to students.* In some variations of true–false items, students correct false statements; for this type, the teacher should award two points, one for identifying the statement as false, and the second point for correcting it. In another variation of true–false items, students supply a rationale for their answers, either true or false. A similar scoring principle might be used in which students receive one point for correctly identifying the answer as true or false and a second point for the rationale.

Sample items follow:

For each of the following statements, circle T if the statement is true and F if the statement is false.

Ⓣ   F   Insulin-dependent diabetes mellitus is also known as Type I
              diabetes. (T)

Ⓣ   F   Hypothyroidism is manifested by lethargy and fatigue. (T)

T   Ⓕ   The most common form of congenital heart defect in child-
              ren is Tetralogy of Fallot. (F)

Variations of True–False Items

There are many variations of true–false items that may be used for testing. One variation is to ask students to correct false statements. Students may identify the words that make a statement false and insert words to make it true. In changing the false statement to a true one, students may write in their own corrections or choose words from a list supplied by the teacher (Bott, 1996). One other modification of true-false items is to have students include a rationale for their responses whether they be true or false, providing a means of testing their comprehension of the content. For all of these variations, the directions should be clear and specific. Some examples follow:

> If the statement is true, draw a circle around T and do no more. If the statement is false, draw a circle around F and underline the word or phrase that makes it false.
>
> T F Tetany occurs with increased secretion of parathyroid hormones.

Since this statement is false, the student would circle F and underline the word "increased":

> T Ⓕ Tetany occurs with <u>increased</u> secretion of parathyroid hormones. (F)

> If the statement is true, draw a circle around T and do no more. If the statement is false, draw a circle around F, underline the word or phrase that makes it false, and write in the blank the word or phrase that would make it true.
>
> T F Canned soups are high in potassium.
>
> _____
>
> T F Fresh fruits and vegetables are low in sodium.
>
> _____

In the first example, because the statement is false, the student would circle F, underline "potassium," and write "sodium" in the blank to make the statement true. In the second example, because the statement is true, the student would only circle T:

> T Ⓕ Canned soups are high in <u>potassium</u>. (F)
>
> Sodium _____
>
> Ⓣ F Fresh fruits and vegetables are low in sodium. (T)
>
> _____

> If the statement is true, draw a circle around T and do no more. If the statement is false, draw a circle around F and circle the *correct* word from the list that follows the item.
>
> T F Bradycardia is a heart rate less than <u>80</u> beats per minute.
>   40, 50, 60, 100

Because the statement is false, the student would circle both F and 60:

T   Ⓕ   Bradycardia is a heart rate less than <u>80</u> beats per minute. (F)
              40, 50, ⑥⓪ 100

If the statement is true, draw a circle around T and explain why it is true. If the statement is false, draw a circle around F and explain why it is false.

Ⓣ   F   Patients with emphysema should have low flow oxygen. (T)

_____

_____

One other variation of true–false items is cluster true–false. Bott (1996) described this as an incomplete statement followed by several phrases to complete it. Students then indicate the phrases which form true or false statements. This type of item resembles multiple-choice questions, if only one phrase completes the statement, or multiple-response, if more than one phrase is true. Ebel and Frisbie (1991) described this variation as a multiple true–false item. Each of the phrases represents a separate true-false statement. One advantage to using this type of question is that students can answer more cluster true-false questions than multiple-choice in a given time frame, enabling the teacher to test more content (Ebel & Frisbie, 1991, p. 151). Directions for answering these items should be clear, and phrases should be numbered consecutively since they represent individual true-false items. Sample items follow:

The incomplete statements below are followed by several phrases. Each of the phrases completes the statement and makes it true or false. If the completed statement is true, draw a circle around T. If the completed statement is false, draw a circle around F.
A patient with a below-the-knee amputation should:

T   Ⓕ   1. avoid walking until fitted with the prosthesis. (F)
T   Ⓕ   2. keep the stump elevated at all times. (F)
Ⓣ   F   3. lift weights to build up arm strength. (T)
Ⓣ   F   4. wrap the stump in a figure-eight style. (T)

Bloom's taxonomy of the cognitive domain includes the:
Ⓣ   F   5. Application level. (T)
Ⓣ   F   6. Knowledge level. (T)
T   Ⓕ   7. Calculation level. (F)

T (F)   8. Recommended actions level. (F)
(T) F   9. Analysis level. (T)
T (F)   10. Manipulation level. (F)
(T) F   11. Synthesis level. (T)

MATCHING

Matching exercises consist of two parallel columns in which students match terms, phrases, sentences, or numbers from one column to the other. One column includes a list of premises and the other column, from which the selection is made, is referred to as responses. The basis for matching responses to premises should be stated explicitly in the directions with the exercise. The student identifies pairs based on the principle specified in these directions. With some matching exercises differences between the premises and responses are not apparent, such as matching a list of laboratory studies with their normal ranges, and the columns could be interchanged. In other exercises, however, the premises include descriptive phrases or sentences to which the student matches shorter responses.

Matching exercises lend themselves to testing categories, classifications, groupings, definitions, and other related facts. They are most appropriate for recall of specific information (Ebel & Frisbie, 1991; Gronlund & Linn, 1990; Reilly & Oermann, 1990). One advantage of a matching exercise is its ability to test a number of facts that can be grouped together rather than designing a series of individual questions. For instance, the teacher can develop one matching exercise on medications and related side effects rather than a series of individual items on each medication. A disadvantage, however, is the focus on recall of facts and specific information although in many courses this reflects an important outcome of learning.

Writing Matching Exercises

Matching exercises are intended for categories, classifications, and information which can be grouped in some way. An effective exercise requires use of homogeneous material with responses which are plausible for multiple premises. Responses that are not plausible for some premises provide clues to the correct match. Principles for writing matching exercises include:

1. *The premises and responses to be matched should be homogeneous,* all concerned with the same content.

2. *Include an unequal number of premises and responses* to avoid giving a clue to the final match. Typically, more responses than premises are included. Ebel and Frisbie (1991) suggest using a list of three premises and

five responses. Others recommend a somewhat longer list ranging from 5 to 12 responses in each matching exercise (Bott, 1996) and up to 15 (Hopkins et al., 1990). With this large number, however, it is difficult to review the choices and pair them with the premises and impossible to record answers on machine-scored answer sheets. For matching exercises with a large number of responses, the teacher might develop two separate matching questions.

3. *Directions for matching exercises should be clear* and state explicitly the basis for matching the premises and responses. This is an important principle in developing these items. Even if the basis for matching seems self-evident, the directions should include the rationale for matching the columns. If responses may be used more than once, the directions should specify this for the learner.

4. *Place the longer premises on the left and shorter responses on the right* (Nitko, 1996). This enables students to read the longer statement first, then search for the correct response, often a single word or few words, on the right. This arrangement saves time and makes the selection easier for students (Bott, 1996). Bott also recommends recording answers on the left side of the page or on a separate answer sheet (p. 130).

5. *The order in which the premises and responses are listed should be alphabetical, numerical, or some other logical order.* Alphabetical order eliminates clues as to the pairing of premises and responses (Ebel & Frisbie, 1991). If the lists have a logical order, however, such as dates and other sequences, then they should be organized in that order. Numbers, quantities, and other related types of items should be arranged in decreasing or increasing order.

6. *The entire matching item should be typed on the same page* and not divided across pages.

Sample matching items follow:

Directions: For each definition in Column A, select the proper term in Column B. Use each letter only once or not at all.

Column A (Premises)	Column B (Responses)
_b_ 1. Attaching a particular response to a specific stimulus	a. Cognitive styles
_f_ 2. Believing that one can respond effectively in a situation	b. Conditioning
	c. Empowerment
_g_ 3. Changing gradually behavioral patterns	d. Modeling
_d_ 4. Observing a behavior and its consequences and attempting to behave similarly	e. Self-care
	f. Self-efficacy
_a_ 5. Varying ways in which individuals process information	g. Shaping

Directions: For each insulin in Column A, identify its peak action in Column B. Responses in Column B may be used once, more than once, or not at all.

Column A	Column B
c 1. Humulin regular	a. Long acting
b 2. NPH	b. Intermediate acting
a 3. PZI	c. Short acting
a 4. Ultralente	

SHORT-ANSWER

Short-answer items, also referred to as completion and fill-in-the-blank, consist of a statement with a key word or words missing or a question to be answered. Students then fill in the blank to complete the statement or answer a question. Gronlund and Linn (1990) differentiated short-answer from completion items. Short-answer items ask a question which the student answers in the blank space; completion items, on the other hand, consist of an incomplete statement that the student completes (p. 143). Either way, the student is asked to record a short answer in the space provided. The statements or questions may stand alone and have no relationship to one another, or may be a series of items in a similar content area.

Because students supply the answers, this type of item reduces the chance of guessing; in addition, calculations may be included for the teacher to review. For this reason completion items have a high discriminating power; students either know or do not know the answer (Bott, 1996, p. 106).

Short-answer items are appropriate for recall of facts and specific information. These items are particularly effective for measuring student ability to interpret data, use formulas correctly, complete calculations, and solve mathematical-type problems. Questions may ask students to label a diagram, name anatomical parts, identify various instruments, and label other types of drawings, photographs, and the like. Bott (1996) describes a controlled completion item as one in which the teacher provides a list of possible responses from which the student selects an answer to complete the blank.

Although completion items appear easy to construct, they should be designed in such a way that only one answer is possible. If students provide other correct answers, the teacher needs to accept them.

Writing Short-Answer Items

Suggestions for developing short-answer items follow:

1. *Statements for students to complete and questions for them to answer should not be quoted directly from textbooks, other readings, and lecture notes.* These materials may be used as a basis for designing short-answer items, but taking statements from them verbatim may result in testing meaningless facts out of context. Such items require memorization of content and may or may not be accompanied by student comprehension of it.

2. *Phrase the item so a unique word, series of words, or number may be supplied to complete it.* Only one correct answer should be possible in response to the question or to complete the statement. The question "What is insulin?" does not provide sufficient direction as to how to respond; asking instead "What is the peak action of NPH insulin?" results in a more specific answer. Before writing the item, think of the correct answer first, then write a question or statement for this answer. Although the goal is developing an item with only one correct response, students may identify other correct answers. For this reason, develop a scoring sheet with all possible correct answers and re-score student responses as needed.

3. *Short-answer items requiring calculations and solving mathematical-type problems should include in the statement the type of answer desired,* for instance, "Convert pounds to kilograms."

4. *For a statement with a key word or words missing, place the blank at the end of the statement.* This makes it easier for students to complete. At the same time, it is important to watch for grammatical clues in the statement, such as "a" versus "an" and singular versus plural, prior to the blank which might give clues to the intended response. If more than one blank is included in the statement, the blanks should be of equal lengths.

5. *If the completion item requires a list, the facts to be supplied should be short,* and able to be expressed in a few words (Bott, 1996). Requiring students to provide long lists of answers takes time and lends itself to more difficulty in terms of scoring. Bott (1996) recommends limiting such lists to six to eight facts only. If the list demands a particular order, the teacher should plan for this scoring prior to testing, for instance, determining how points will be deducted for items on the list that are correct but out of order.

6. *When students need to write in longer answers, provide for sufficient space* or use a separate answer sheet.

7. *Even though a blank space should be placed at the end of the statement, the teacher may direct the student to record one-word answers in blanks arranged in a column* to the left or right of the items, thereby facilitating scoring. For example,

_____1. *Streptococcus pneumoniae* and *Staphylococcus aureus* are examples of _____ bacteria.

Sample short-answer items follow:

Two types of meter-dose inhalers used for the treatment of bronchial asthma are: _____
_____

What congenital cardiac defect results in communication between the pulmonary artery and aorta? _____

List the five phases of Doherty and Campbell's family health and illness cycle in the order in which they occur.

_____
_____
_____
_____
_____

SUMMARY

Test items may be categorized broadly as objective and essay. Objective items, which are structured and ask the student to supply an answer or choose among alternatives, include true–false, matching, short-answer, multiple-choice, and multiple-response. Essay questions provide an opportunity for students to formulate their own ideas and express them in writing. In addition to these, there are many other types of evaluation methods appropriate for assessing student learning in nursing courses and clinical practice.

This chapter introduced objective tests and described how to construct three types of test items: true–false, matching, and short answer, and variations on them. Suggestions for writing these items and sample questions also were included.

A true–false item consists of a statement that the student judges as true or false. Each item represents a declarative sentence stating a fact or principle and asks the learner to decide if it is true or false, right or wrong, or correct or incorrect. In some forms, students correct a response or supply a rationale as to why the statement is true or false. True–false items are most effective for recall of facts and specific information, but also may be used to test the student's comprehension of an important principle or concept.

Matching exercises consist of two parallel columns in which students match terms, phrases, sentences, or numbers from one column to the other. One column includes a list of premises and the other column, from which the selection is made, is referred to as responses. The student identifies pairs based on the principle specified in the directions. Matching exercises lend themselves to testing categories, classifications, groupings, definitions, and other related facts. Similar to true–false, they are most appropriate for recall of specific information.

Short-answer items consist of a statement with a key word or words missing or a question to be answered. Students then fill in the blank to complete the statement or answer a question. Short-answer items are appropriate for recall of facts and specific information. These items are particularly effective for measuring student ability to interpret data, use formulas correctly, complete calculations, and solve mathematical-type problems.

In developing an evaluation protocol, the teacher has multiple types of test items and evaluation strategies from which to choose. Two other types of objective items, multiple-choice and multiple-response, are described in chapter 5.

REFERENCES

Bott, P. A. (1996). *Testing and assessment in occupational and technical education*. Boston: Allyn and Bacon.

Ebel, R. L., & Frisbie, D. A. (1991). *Essentials of educational measurement* (5th ed.). Englewood Cliffs, NJ: Prentice Hall.

Gronlund, N. E., & Linn, R. L. (1990). *Measurement and evaluation in teaching* (6th ed.). New York: Macmillan.

Hopkins, K. D., Stanley, J. C., & Hopkins, B. R. (1990). *Educational and psychological measurement and evaluation* (7th ed.). Englewood Cliffs, NJ: Prentice Hall.

Kubiszyn, T., & Borich, G. (1993). *Educational testing and measurement* (4th ed.). New York: Harper Collins.

Nitko, A. J. (1996). *Educational assessment of students* (2nd ed.). Englewood Cliffs, NJ: Prentice Hall.

Reilly, D. E., & Oermann, M. H. (1990). *Behavioral objectives: Evaluation in nursing* (3rd ed.). New York: National League for Nursing.

5

Objective Test Items: Multiple-Choice and Multiple-Response

Multiple-choice and multiple-response are the other two types of objective items. Multiple-choice items, with one correct answer, are used widely in nursing and other fields. This format of test item includes an incomplete statement or question, followed by a list of options that complete the statement or answer the question. Multiple-response items are designed similarly, although more than one answer may be correct. Both of these formats of test items may be used for evaluating learning at the recall, comprehension, application, and analysis levels, making them adaptable for a wide range of content and learning outcomes.

MULTIPLE-CHOICE ITEMS

Gronlund and Linn (1990) identified three broad uses of multiple-choice items:

1. *to measure knowledge* of terms, specific facts, principles, and methods;
2. *to examine student comprehension* of the content; and
3. *to measure ability* to apply facts and principles, interpret cause-and-effect relationships, and justify methods and procedures.

Other uses of multiple-choice testing include: definitions; understanding of relationships between two or more actions or phenomena (Bott, 1996); application of concepts and theories in care; analysis of data, client status, and clinical situations; comparisons of varied interventions; and judgments and decisions regarding actions to take with clients and families. Multiple-choice items are useful for testing application of nursing knowledge in simulated clinical situations. Bloom, Englehart, Furst, Hill, and Krathwohl (1956) indicated that measurement of learning at the application level required use of knowledge in a *new* situation. The multiple-choice format provides an opportunity for the teacher to introduce new clinical situations requiring application of concepts and theories or analytical thinking in order to respond to the questions. Multiple-choice is the predominant format used for testing in nursing not only in terms of teacher-made tests, but also for licensing, certification, and other commercially available examinations.

Although there are many advantages to multiple-choice testing, there also are disadvantages. First, these items are difficult to construct, particularly at the higher cognitive levels. Developing items to test memorization of facts is much easier than designing ones to measure use of knowledge in a new situation and skill in analysis. As such, many multiple-choice items are written at the lower cognitive levels, focusing only on recall and comprehension. Second, teachers often experience difficulty developing plausible, yet incorrect, distracters. If the distracters are not plausible, a clue is provided to omit that possibility. Third, it is often difficult to identify only one correct answer. For these reasons, multiple-choice items are time-consuming to construct.

Some critics of objective testing suggest that essay and related types of questions that require students to develop a response provide a truer measure of learning than objective testing, in which students typically choose from available options. Ebel and Frisbie (1991) disagreed with this assumption and noted the complexity of thinking often required for making such a selection. They also pointed out that selecting the correct answer in a multiple-choice item requires comparative judgments of the alternatives (p. 157).

Writing Multiple-Choice Items

There are three parts in a multiple-choice item, each with its own set of principles for development: (a) stem, (b) answer, and (c) distracters. The stem is the lead-in phrase in the form of a question or incomplete statement that relies on the alternatives for completion. Following the stem is a list of alternatives, options for the learner to consider and choose from. These alternatives are of two types: the answer, which is the correct or best alternative to answer the question or complete the statement, and distracters, which are the incorrect alternatives. The distracters are to *distract* students who are unsure of the correct answer. Suggestions for writing each of these parts are considered separately.

STEM

The stem is the question or incomplete statement to which the alternatives relate. Gronlund and Linn (1990) suggested that writing the stem in a question form is easier than an incomplete statement; when a statement is preferred, they recommend first developing it as a direct question, then converting the question to an incomplete statement. Suggestions follow for writing the stem.

1. *The stem should present clearly and explicitly the problem to be solved.* After reading the stem, the learner should know what to look for in the alternatives. Chenevey (1988) indicated that this clarity enables the student to "anticipate the correct response even before reading the options" (p. 203). The stem should provide sufficient information for answering the question or completing the statement. An example of this principle follows:

Cataracts:
  a. are painful.
  b. may accompany coronary artery disease.
  c. occur with aging.*
  d. result in tunnel vision.

The stem of this question does not present clearly the problem associated with cataracts that the alternatives address. As such, it does not guide the learner in reviewing the alternatives. In addition, the options are dissimilar, which is possibly due to the lack of clarity in the stem; alternatives should be similar in nature. One possible revision of this item is:

Causes of cataracts include:
  a. aging.*
  b. arteriosclerosis.
  c. hemorrhage.
  d. iritis.

Cover the alternatives and read the stem alone. Does it explain the problem and direct the learner to the alternatives? Is it complete? Could it stand alone as a short-answer item? In writing the stem, always include the nature of the response, such as, Which of the following *interventions, signs and symptoms, treatments, data,* and so forth. A stem that asks, Which of the following? does not provide clear instructions as to what to look for in the options.

2. *Although the stem should be clear and explicit, it should not contain extraneous information* unless the item is developed for the purpose of identifying significant versus insignificant data. Otherwise, the stem should be brief, including only necessary information. Long options that include irrelevant information take additional time for reading. This point can be illustrated using the above example:

> Mrs. J is a new client through the home health agency. She lives alone, although her daughter visits frequently. Mrs. J has congestive heart failure and some shortness of breath. She was told recently that she has cataracts. Causes of cataracts include:
> a. aging.*
> b. arteriosclerosis.
> c. hemorrhage.
> d. iritis.

In this stem, the background information about Mrs. J is irrelevant to the problem addressed. If subsequent items were written about the patient's other problems, related nursing interventions, the home setting, and so forth, then the stem might remain long and detailed. Otherwise, the stem should be as concise as possible.

3. *Avoid inserting information in the stem for instructional purposes.* For instance:

> Cataracts are an opacity of the lens or capsule of the eye leading to blurred and eventual loss of vision. Causes of cataracts include:
> a. aging.*
> b. arteriosclerosis.
> c. hemorrhage.
> d. iritis.

The definition of "cataract" has no relevance to the content tested, that is, causes of cataracts. Ebel and Frisbie (1991) referred to these as "instructional insertions," cautioning teachers to avoid them and focus instead on the content to be evaluated (p. 162).

4. *If words need to be repeated in each alternative to complete the statement, shift them to the stem.* This is illustrated as follows:

An early and common sign of pregnancy:
a. *is* amenorrhea.*
b. *is* morning sickness.
c. *is* spotting.
d. *is* tenderness of the breasts.

The word "is" may be moved to the stem:

An early and common sign of pregnancy *is*:
a. amenorrhea.*
b. morning sickness.
c. spotting.
d. tenderness of the breasts.

Similarly, a word or phrase repeated in each alternative does not test students' knowledge of it and should be included in the stem. An example follows:

Clinical manifestations of Parkinson's disease include:
a. decreased perspiration, tremors at rest, and *muscle rigidity.**
b. increased salivation, *muscle rigidity*, and diplopia.
c. *muscle rigidity*, decreased salivation, and nystagmus.
d. tremors during activity, *muscle rigidity*, and increased perspiration.

This item does not test knowledge of muscle rigidity occurring with Parkinson's disease because it is included with each alternative. The stem could be revised as follows:

Clinical manifestations of Parkinson's disease include *muscle rigidity* and which of the following signs and symptoms?
a. Decreased salivation and nystagmus
b. Increased salivation and diplopia
c. Tremors at rest and decreased perspiration*
d. Tremors during activity and increased perspiration

5. *Do not include key words in the stem that would clue the student to the correct answer.* This point may be demonstrated in the earlier question on cataracts.

Mrs. J is an *elderly* client who lives alone. She was told recently that she has cataracts. Causes of cataracts include:

a. aging.*
b. arteriosclerosis.
c. hemorrhage.
d. iritis.

In this question, informing the student that Mrs. J is elderly provides a clue to the correct response.

6. *Avoid the use of negatively stated stems,* such as "no," "not," and "except." Most stems may be stated positively, asking students for the correct or best response rather than the exception. Negatively stated stems are sometimes unclear; in addition, they require a change in thought pattern from selections that represent correct and best responses to ones reflecting incorrect and least likely responses. If a negatively stated stem is used, however, highlight this for the learner by underlining or capitalizing the negative word or using bold text. Otherwise, words such as "no," "not," and "except" may be overlooked in reading the stem. A sample item follows:

You are working in an agency that cares for the chronically mentally ill in their homes. One of your patients is readmitted after refusing to take her medications. A highly structured routine is used with the goal of preparing her for discharge. All of the following outcomes suggest that this plan is effective *EXCEPT*:

a. asking the nurse for assistance in dressing.*
b. attending occupational therapy on the unit.
c. going to the cafeteria for meals without prompting.
d. telling another patient to move out of "her" chair.

7. *The stem and alternatives that follow should be consistent grammatically.* If the stem is an incomplete statement, each option should complete it grammatically; if not, clues are provided as to the correct or incorrect responses. Along a similar line, check carefully that a consistent verb tense is used with the alternatives. An example follows:

Mrs. S is undergoing a right carotid endarterectomy. Prior to surgery, which information would be most important to collect as a baseline for the early recovery period? Her ability to:

a. follow movements with her eyes.
b. move all four extremities.*
c. rota*ting* her head from side to side.
d. swallow and gag.

Option "c" provides a grammatical clue by not completing the statement, "Her ability to . . ." The item may be revised easily:

Mrs. S is undergoing a right carotid endarterectomy. Prior to surgery, which information would be most important to collect as a baseline for the early recovery period? Her ability to:
a. follow movements with her eyes.
b. move all four extremities.*
c. rotate her head from side to side.
d. swallow and gag.

8. *Avoid ending stems with "a" or "an"*; these may provide grammatical clues as to the options to select. Rephrase the stem to eliminate the "a/an." For instance,

Narrowing of the aortic valve in children occurs with *an*:
a. aortic stenosis.*
b. atrial septal defect.
c. coarctation of the aorta.
d. patent ductus arteriosus.

Ending this stem with "an" eliminates alternatives "c" and "d" because of grammatical errors. The stem could be rewritten by deleting the "an":

Narrowing of the aortic valve in children occurs with:
a. aortic stenosis.*
b. atrial septal defect.
c. coarctation of the aorta.
d. patent ductus arteriosus.

9. *If the stem is a statement completed by the alternatives, begin each alternative with a lower-case letter and place a period after it,* since it forms a sentence with the stem. At the end of the stem, use a comma or colon as appropriate. Use upper-case letters to begin alternatives that do not form a sentence with the stem. If the stem is a question, place a question mark at the end.

10. *Each multiple-choice item should be independent of the others.* This principle holds true except for multiple-choice items that are developed in a series, with a number of items that relate to one client situation or a common data set. In a series of items, the directions should indicate that questions _____ to _____ pertain to the scenario. A sample item follows illustrating questions that are not meant to stand alone.

Directions: Questions 1 and 2 relate to the following client situation. Select the best answer in each of these questions.
Mr. G is a 45-year-old male who was treated in the ER for an asthma attack.

1. You are the community health nurse developing his teaching plan. Which action should be implemented *FIRST*?
   a. Assess other related health problems.
   b. Determine his level of understanding of asthma.*
   c. Review with him treatments for his asthma.
   d. Teach him actions of his medications.

2. On your second home visit, Mr. G is short of breath. Which of these statements indicates a need for further instruction?
   a. "I checked my peak flow since I'm not feeling good."
   b. "I have been turning on the air conditioner at times like this."
   c. "I tried my Azmacort because my chest was feeling heavy."*
   d. "I used my nebulizer mist treatment for my wheezing."

11. *Write the stem so that the alternatives are placed at the end of the incomplete statement.* Bott (1996) suggested that an incomplete statement with a blank in the middle, which the options then complete, is confusing for students to read and follow.

ANSWER

Following the stem in a multiple-choice item is a list of alternatives, including the correct, or best, answer and distracters. There are varying proposals as to the number of alternatives to include with an item, ranging from three to five. Gronlund and Linn (1991) indicated that five choices reduce the chance of guessing the correct answer to one in five. The larger the number of alternatives, if plausible, the more discriminating the item (Ebel & Frisbie, 1990). Unfortunately, it is difficult to develop four plausible distracters to accompany the correct answer when five options are included. For this reason, typically four choices are used, allowing for one correct or best answer and three plausible distracters.

In some instances the best, rather than correct, answer is selected from the alternatives. Considering that judgments are needed to arrive at decisions about client care, often items are designed for the student to judge the best or most appropriate response from those listed. Best answers are valuable for more complex and higher level learning, such as with questions written at the application and analysis levels. According to Bott

(1996), best-answer items require inferential reasoning and a complete understanding of the concept to select the best option.

If there is a correct answer, Ebel and Frisbie (1991) recommended that this be used, rather than the best answer. Teachers "should not settle for a best answer when a correct one to the same question is available" (p. 166). Regardless of whether the correct or best answer format is used, the item needs to be written so that only one answer is appropriate. When it is the best answer, there should be consistency in the literature and among experts as to this response.

Suggestions for writing the correct answer are:

1. *Review the alternatives carefully to assure that there is only one correct response.* For example:

Symptoms of increased intracranial pressure include:
   a. blurred vision.*
   b. decreased blood pressure.
   c. disorientation.*
   d. increased pulse.

In this sample item, both "a" and "c" are correct; a possible revision follows:

Symptoms of increased intracranial pressure include:
   a. blurred vision and decreased blood pressure.
   b. decreased blood pressure and increased pulse.
   c. disorientation and blurred vision.*
   d. increased pulse and disorientation.

2. *Carefully review terminology included in the stem* to avoid giving a clue to the correct answer. Key words in the stem, if also used in the correct response, may clue the student to select it. In the following example, "sudden weight loss" is in both the stem and answer:

An elderly patient is seen in the clinic with *sudden weight loss*, thirst, and confusion. Which of the following signs would be indicative of dehydration?
   a. Below normal temperature
   b. Decreased urine-specific gravity
   c. Increased blood pressure
   d. *Sudden weight loss**

The question could be revised by omitting "sudden weight loss" in the stem:

> An elderly patient is seen in the clinic with dry skin, thirst, and confusion. Which of the following signs also would be indicative of dehydration?
> a. Below normal temperature
> b. Decreased urine-specific gravity
> c. Increased blood pressure
> d. *Sudden weight loss**

3. *The alternatives should be similar in length, detail, and complexity and should sample the same domain of knowledge;* for instance, all symptoms, all diagnostic studies, all nursing interventions, varying treatments, and so forth. Check the number of words included in each option for consistency in length. Frequently the correct answer is the longest as the teacher attempts to write it clearly and specifically. Nitko (1996) explained that the test-wise student may realize that the longest response is the correct answer without having the requisite knowledge to make this choice. In this case, either shorten the correct response or add similar qualifiers to the distracters, so that they are similar in length as well as detail and complexity.

Although there is no established number of words by which the alternatives may differ from each other without providing clues, count the words in each option and attempt to vary them by no more than a few words. This will provide a check that the options are consistent in length. The student should not identify the correct response and eliminate distracters because of the way in which they are written. In the sample item, the correct answer is longer than the distracters, which might provide a clue to select it.

> You are assessing a 14-year-old girl who appears emaciated. Her mother describes the following changes: resistance to eating and 20-lb. weight loss over the last 6 weeks. It is most likely that the client resists eating for which of the following reasons?
> a. Complains of recurring nausea
> b. Describes herself as "fat all over" and fearful of gaining weight*
> c. Has other GI problems
> d. Seeks her mother's attention

The correct answer can be shortened to: "Is fearful of gaining weight."
In addition to consistency in length, detail, and complexity, the correct

response should contain the same number of parts as the distracters. The answer in the previous question is not only longer than the other options, but also includes two parts, providing another clue. In developing alternatives, attempt to include the same number of parts in each option. In the example that follows, including two causes in option "a" provides a clue as to the correct response. Revising this option to include aging only avoids this.

Causes of cataracts include:
a. aging and steroid therapy.*
b. arteriosclerosis.
c. hemorrhage.
d. iritis.

4. *The alternatives should be consistent grammatically.* Use similar structure and terminology for the answer and other options. Avoid including opposite responses, as this often clues the student to choose between these two and omit consideration of the other options. A sample item follows:

The nurse determines the correct placement of a nasogastric tube by:
a. asking the patient to swallow.
b. inserting water in the tube and auscultating in the epigastric area.
c. inserting air in the tube and auscultating in the epigastric area.*
d. taping the tube in place and checking it.

In this example, the correct response is opposite one of the distracters, clueing the student to select one of these options. In addition, options "b" and "c" begin with "inserting" that may provide a visual clue to choose between them. Option "a" contains one part, in contrast to the other alternatives.

5. *The correct answer should be randomly assigned to a position among the alternatives* to avoid favoring a particular response choice, for instance, a tendency to assign the correct answer to the "c" option. Gaberson (1996) recommended that the alternatives be arranged in a logical or meaningful order, such as alphabetical or chronological. Options reflecting size or degree should be arranged sequentially, either increasing or decreasing in value. This in turn tends to randomly distribute the position of the correct response throughout the test. It also helps students locate the correct response more easily when they have an answer in mind.

6. *Answers should not reflect the opinion of the teacher,* but instead should represent the most probable response or one accepted by experts in the subject area (Ebel & Frisbie, 1991; Nitko, 1996).

DISTRACTERS

Distracters are the incorrect although plausible alternatives. The purpose of the distracter is to "distract" the student who is unsure of the correct response. Distracters should appeal to learners who lack the knowledge for responding to the question. If the option is obviously wrong, then there is no reason to include it as an alternative. Each distracter should be selected by some students, and if not, it should be revised for future tests. In writing distracters, think about common errors students make; phrases that "sound correct"; misperceptions students have regarding the content; words associated with the stem, such as managerial and manager; and familiar responses not appropriate for the specific problem. Ebel and Frisbie (1991) provided strategies for developing effective distracters:

- Define a group or category to which all alternative responses must belong. For instance, if the stem asks about side effects of ery- thromycin, then plausible distracters may be drawn from side effects of antibiotics as a group.
- Consider content that has some association with the terms used in the stem. If the question deals with oxygen therapy for a patient with COPD, consider other conditions requiring different types of oxygen therapy.
- If the answer is quantitative, the distracters should be points along the same scale, such as varying blood pressures, temperatures, weights, and so forth.
- If unable to identify plausible distracters that are consistent with the stem, then consider rewriting the stem (pp. 168–170).

Suggestions for writing distracters include:

1. *The distracters and correct answer should be consistent grammatically; should be similar in length, detail, and complexity; and should sample the same domain of knowledge.* Check that distracters are written with the same speci- ficity as the correct response.

2. *Each alternative should be appropriate for completing the stem.* Hastily written distracters may be clearly incorrect, different in substance and for- mat from the others, and inappropriate for the stem, providing clues as to how to respond and not measuring students' learning.

3. *Options with numbers, quantities, and other numerical values should be listed sequentially,* either increasing or decreasing in value, and should not overlap. An example of this principle is:

Compressions for infant CPR should be:

a. $1^1/_2$ to 2 inches.
b. $^1/_4$ to $^1/_2$ inch.
c. $^1/_2$ to 1 inch.*
d. 1 to 2 inches.

The values in these options overlap, such as with "a" and "d"; "b" and "c"; and "c" and "d." They would be easier to review if arranged sequentially from decreasing to increasing length. A revision follows:

Compressions for infant CPR should be:

a. Less than $^1/_8$ inch.
b. $^1/_8$ to $^1/_4$ inch.
c. $^1/_2$ to 1 inch.*
d. $1^1/_2$ to 2 inches.

4. *Avoid using "all of the above" and "none of the above" in a multiple-choice item.* As distracters these are in contrast to the direction of selecting one correct or best response. With "all of the above" as a distracter, students aware of one incorrect response are clued to eliminate "all of the above" as an option. Along a similar line, knowledge of one correct response clues students to omit "none of the above" as an option. Ebel and Frisbie (1991) and Nitko (1996), however, expressed a different point of view in terms of these options. They suggested that "all of the above" is appropriate as an option if all of the alternatives are correct answers to the stem. Kubiszyn and Borich (1993), though, indicated that "all of the above" is typically the correct answer, making the item too easy. "None of the above" is appropriate only with correct answer-type questions, not when students are asked to choose the best response (Gronlund & Linn, 1990; Kubiszyn & Borich, 1993; Nitko, 1996).

5. *In most instances terms such as "always," "never," "sometimes," "occasionally," and other similar ones should be omitted from the distracters;* they may provide clues as to the correctness of the option.

6. *Avoid using distracters that are essentially the same.* For example:

A student comes to see the school nurse complaining of a severe headache and stiff neck. Which of the following actions would be most appropriate?

a. Ask the student to rest in the clinic for a few hours.
b. Collect additional data before deciding on interventions.*
c. Have a family member take the student home to rest.
d. Prepare to take the student to the emergency room.

Alternatives "a" and "c" are essentially the same; if "rest" is eliminated as an option, learners are clued to omit both of these. In addition, the correct response in this item is more general than the others and not specific to this particular student's health problems. The item could be revised as follows:

A student comes to see the school nurse complaining of a severe headache and stiff neck. Which of the following actions would be most appropriate?
a. Ask the student to rest in the clinic for a few hours.
b. Check the student's health record for identified health problems.*
c. Prepare to take the student to the emergency room.
d. Send the student back to class after medicating for pain.

7. *Each option should be placed on a separate line for ease of student reading.* If answers are recorded on a separate answer sheet, review the format of the sheet ahead of time so responses are identified as "a" through "d" or 1 through 4 as appropriate.

Analogy-Type Multiple-Choice

Bott (1996) described a variation of multiple-choice items relating to analogies that might be incorporated within nursing tests. In analogy-type items, the student identifies the relationship that exists between the first two parts of an item, then uses it for selecting the correct response (pp. 90–91). An illustration of this type of item follows:

Directions: In the items that follow, identify the relationship that exists between the first two words, then use this relationship to select the correct option. The first item is included as an example:
 b 1. Describe is to comprehension as awareness is to:
        a. imitation.
        b. receiving.*
        c. responding.
        d. valuing.

___ 2. Orem is to self-care as Roy is to:
        a. adaptation.*
        b. care.
        c. client system.
        d. transaction.

___ 3. Lasix is to diuretic as Inderal is to:
   a. adrenergic inhibitor.*
   b. antiarrhythmic.
   c. calcium blocker.
   d. vasodilator.

Testing in Nursing Process Framework

As students progress through a nursing program, they develop abilities to assess clients with varied needs and health problems, analyze data and derive multiple nursing diagnoses, set realistic goals for care considering the demands within the health care system, critique nursing interventions and select appropriate ones, and evaluate the effectiveness of care. Multiple-choice testing within the framework of the nursing process provides an opportunity to measure this learning. Items may be written about phases of the nursing process, decisions to be made in clinical situations and consequences of each, varying judgments possible in a situation, and other questions which examine students' critical thinking ability as related to the situation described in the test item. This type of testing provides a means of evaluating higher and more complex levels of learning. Questions may be written at the application and analysis levels, examining student ability to apply concepts and theories to the situation described in the item and engage in analytical thinking to arrive at an answer. This format of multiple-choice testing also provides experience for students in answering the types of questions encountered in the National Council Licensure Examination for Registered Nurses (NCLEX–RN).

Current practices suggest that often multiple-choice items are developed at the recall and comprehension levels and not at higher levels of learning. Evaluating ability to apply concepts and analyze situations is important particularly as students progress through the nursing program and for evaluation of nurses in practice. In addition to a preponderance of lower level questions, teachers often focus questions on scientific rationale, principles related to care, and selection of interventions. Fewer questions are developed on collecting and analyzing data; determining nursing diagnoses; setting realistic goals of care; and evaluating client progress, the effectiveness of interventions, delivery of care, and other outcomes. Testing within a nursing process framework provides an opportunity to develop these types of test questions.

NCLEX–RN

The intent of this section of the chapter is not to describe the development of the nursing licensing examination; some discussion is provided, however, to place this type of testing within the NCLEX–RN framework.

The NCLEX–RN measures the knowledge, skills, and abilities essential for entry-level practice as a registered nurse (RN). The content to be tested was developed from a 1992–1993 job analysis study of newly licensed entry-level RNs. Job analysis studies delineate the content domain for measuring critical knowledge and skills for safe practice, provide information about the activities RNs perform in their jobs, and serve as a means of validating the licensure examination (Chornick & Yocom, 1995). Passing the test indicates that the nurse has a minimum level of competence to practice as an entry-level RN (Beare, 1995). Licensure examinations are by their nature one way of assuring the public that the professional has sufficient knowledge and skills to deliver safe care.

The test plan includes two major components: (a) phases of the nursing process, including assessment, analysis, planning, implementation, and evaluation; and (b) client needs. Each of the phases of the nursing process carries approximately equal weight, 17–23%. The client needs include safe and effective care environment (15–21% of the items); physiological integrity (46–54%); psychosocial integrity (8–16%); and health promotion and maintenance (17–23%) (National Council of State Boards of Nursing [NCSBN], 1995b). Questions are written at the knowledge, comprehension, application, and analysis levels.

The NCLEX–PN test plan is similar to the NCLEX–RN plan except that only four steps of the nursing process are assessed: collecting data, planning, implementing, and evaluating. In addition, the percentage of items in each client need category differs to reflect practice as a practical/vocational nurse: safe, effective care environment (24–30%); physiological integrity (42–48%); psychosocial integrity (7–13%); and health promotion and maintenance (15–21%) (NCSBN, 1995a, p. 10).

In 1994 the licensing examination changed from a paper-and-pencil format to a computer adaptive test (CAT) model. Research has indicated that both forms of testing are comparable. With the CAT examination, there is a 5-hour maximum amount of time allowed for completion of the items. Two hundred and sixty-five items is the maximum number presented; 75 is the minimum number to be answered (Beare, 1995, p. 33). Fifteen of these questions are tryout items that are unscored (NCSBN, 1996).

The CAT model is such that each candidate's test is assembled interactively as the person is answering the questions. Each item has a predetermined difficulty level. When the item is answered, the computer calculates a skill estimate based on the person's earlier answer and selects from a large data bank an item designed to measure the candidate's ability most precisely (NCSBN, 1994). This process is built upon the Rasch measurement model, an Item Response Theory (IRT) model, that has been used to "equate the difficulty of different sets of NCLEX questions" (NCSBN, 1995a). Using this model, a large set of test questions with known difficulties has been established from which items are drawn for individual candidates. This is an efficient means of testing, avoiding questions that do not contribute to determining a candidate's level of nursing competence. The licensing examination is therefore tailored to the individual's knowledge and skills, yet still measures competence as required by the test plan (NCSBN, 1995a). The standard for passing the NCLEX is criterion-referenced; a passing standard is set by the NCSBN based on an established protocol and used as the basis for determining if the individual has passed or failed the examination.

Research in nursing has examined predictors of success on the NCLEX–RN. While differences exist across studies, some of the variables predicting performance on the NCLEX–RN include high school ranking and standardized test scores such as SAT (Dell & Valine,1990; McKinney, Small, O'Dell, & Coonrod, 1988; Yang, Glick, & McClelland, 1987); standardized tests students take in preparation for the licensing examination, such as Mosby AssessTest (Jenks, Selekman, Bross, & Paquet, 1989; McKinney et al., 1988); prerequisite nursing courses (Payne & Duffey, 1986; Yang et al., 1987); and grades in nursing courses and overall grade point average (Dell & Valine, 1990; Horns, O'Sullivan, & Goodman, 1991; Krupa, Quick, & Whitley, 1988; Lengacher & Keller, 1990; McKinney et al., 1988; Mills, Sampel, Pohlman, & Becker, 1992; Payne & Duffey, 1986). Academic achievement, expressed by nursing course grades and overall grade point average, has been found across studies as predictive of student performance on the NCLEX–RN. Experience with this type of testing within nursing courses prepares students for answering similar questions on the licensing examination. In addition to this format of test items, students also need practice with computer adaptive testing.

A second area of the literature on the NCLEX–RN focuses on strategies for preparing students to pass the examination. Ashley and O'Neil (1994) reported on the effectiveness of faculty-directed study groups as an intervention to prepare candidates for the NCLEX–RN, particularly among students of lower academic achievement. Other educators have examined programs for improving students' verbal and study skills (Foti & DeYoung, 1991); providing individualized study plans for students (Eason & Woolard, 1991); intensive intervention programs (Hussey, Wolahan, & Wieczorek, 1991); and other strategies including practice with computer examinations, teacher-directed NCLEX–RN seminars, content review books and computer programs, flash cards, and other study aids (Beare, 1995).

Writing Nursing Process Items

Nursing process items may be written at the knowledge, comprehension, application, and analysis levels. If the outcome to be tested is recall and comprehension, though, other types of items may be as appropriate, and are typically easier to construct. Nursing process items at the application and analysis levels are more difficult and time-consuming to develop.

In developing items on the nursing process at varying cognitive levels, it is important to remember the outcome of learning intended at each of these levels. Questions at the knowledge level deal with facts, principles, and other specific information related to each phase of the nursing process. At the comprehension level, items measure understanding of concepts and ability to explain them. At the application level, students need to apply concepts and theories as a basis for responding to the item. Reilly and Oermann (1990) explained that at this level, test questions measure use of knowledge in assessment, analysis, planning, intervention, and evaluation. Questions at the analysis level are the most difficult to construct. They require analysis of a client situation to identify critical elements and relationships among them, deriving "meaning from the situation using resources outside of the data at hand" (Reilly & Oermann, 1990, p. 202). Questions should provide a new situation for students to analyze, not one encountered previously for which the student might recall the analysis. The difference between application and analysis items is not always readily apparent; analysis items, though, should require students to identify relevant data, critical elements, component parts, and their interrelationships. This goal is often achieved by describing client situations not encountered previously in practice or discussions, with sufficient detail for the student to analyze.

The process of developing nursing process items begins with identifying the total number of items to be written. This includes specifying the number of questions for each phase of the nursing process. On some tests, greater weight may be given to certain phases of the process, as these were emphasized in the instruction. As part of this planning, the teacher also maps out the clinical situations to be tested as relevant to course content. For instance, the teacher may plan for two assessment questions on pain; three intervention questions, including two on nursing management and a third on medications; and one item on evaluating the effectiveness of pain management with children. A similar process may be used with other content areas for which this type of testing is intended. Questions may stand alone, or a series of items may be developed around one client scenario. In the latter format, the teacher has an option of adding data to the client situation, expanding it for testing purposes.

Test items on assessment examine knowledge of data to collect, use of varied sources of data, relevancy of selected data for a client, verifying data, communicating data, and documenting findings. Analysis questions, referring to the nursing process, not the analysis level in Bloom's taxonomy, measure ability to interpret data, identify client problems and needs, and determine nursing diagnoses. Questions on the planning phase of the nursing process focus on setting realistic goals for individuals, families, and communities; planning nursing measures to achieve outcomes of care; and collaborating with others in developing plans. Questions on implementation relate to the student's understanding of principles underlying varied interventions and their use in the clinical setting; selection of nursing measures for individuals, families, and communities; ability to critique interventions; and documentation of care in varied types of clinical settings. The last phase for which questions may be written is evaluation. These items focus on client responses, the quality dimension of care, the extent to which the outcomes of care have been achieved, variables influencing care delivery, recording client progress and outcomes, and needed revisions of the plan of care based on evaluative data.

Examples of stems that may be used to develop questions for each phase of the nursing process are provided in Table 5.1. These examples are not meant to be exhaustive; instead, they illustrate how stems may be written and provide a guide for teachers to use in developing their own questions. Sample items for each phase of the nursing process follow:

Assessment

Ben, an 8-year-old, is brought to the emergency room by his mother after falling off his bike and hitting his head. Which of the following data are most important to collect in the initial assessment?

a. Blood pressure
b. Level of consciousness
c. Pupillary response
d. Respiratory status*

Analysis

Ms. A is a 17-year-old seen in the clinic for pelvic inflammatory disease. The nurse should anticipate which of the following nursing diagnoses?

a. Altered health maintenance
b. Pain*
c. Knowledge deficit
d. Sexual dysfunction

Table 5.1 Examples of Stems for Nursing Process Questions

Assessment
- The nurse should collect which of the following data?
- Which of the following information should be collected as a priority in the assessment process?
- Which of the following data should be collected first? Now?
- Which of the following questions should be asked by the nurse in assessing the client/family?
- What additional data are needed to establish the nursing diagnosis?
- Which of the following information is most important at this time?
- What resources should be used to collect the data?

Analysis
- These data support the nursing diagnosis of _____.
- Which nursing diagnosis is most appropriate for this client?
- The priority nursing diagnosis is _____.
- The priority health problem of this client/family/community is

    _____.

Planning
- The goal of care for this client is _____.
- Which of the following goals is most important at this time?
- Nursing measures to be included in the plan of care are:
- To achieve the goal/outcome of _____, which nursing intervention(s) should be included in the plan of care?
- Resources to be incorporated in the plan of care for the client include:

Implementation
- Which of the following actions should be implemented immediately?
- Nursing interventions for this client include:
- Referrals for the client/family include:
- Following this procedure/surgery/treatment/test, which nursing measures should be implemented?
- Which of these nursing interventions are essential considering the client's change in health status?
- Teaching for this patient/family includes:
- Which of the following instructions should be given to the patient/family?

Evaluation
- Which of these client responses indicates the nursing interventions are effective?

(continued)

Table 5.1 *(cont.)*

- Which of these responses indicates the treatment/medication/intervention is achieving its desired effect?
- Based on these data, which of the following outcomes of care have been/have not been met?
- Which response indicates improvement in the client's condition?
- The client should be observed for side effects of _____ / responses to _____?
- Which of these statements by the client/family indicates a need for further teaching/an understanding of the instruction?

Note. From *Behavioral Objectives: Evaluation in Nursing* (3rd ed., pp. 203–210), by D. E. Reilly and M. H. Oermann, 1990. New York: National League for Nursing. Copyright 1990 by National League for Nursing. Adapted with permission.

Planning

To facilitate the breathing of a 12-month-old with bronchiolitis, the nursing care plan should include caring for the child in an environment of:
a. cool, moist oxygen.*
b. humidified oxygen.
c. oxygen therapy with no mist.
d. warm mist with oxygen.†

Implementation

A 32-year-old woman was admitted in active labor to labor and delivery. Contractions are every 2 minutes lasting 50 to 60 seconds. She is 6-cm. dilated and 100% effaced, and membranes are intact. The fetal heart rate is 140 and regular, and the client's blood pressure is 80/40. Before checking the BP again, the nurse should *FIRST*:
a. attach an external fetal monitor.
b. call the physician.
c. place her in Trendelenburg's position.
d. turn the client to her left side.†*

Evaluation

Mr. P was discharged following a below-the-knee amputation. You are making the first home health visit after his discharge. Which of the following statements by Mr. P indicates that he needs further instruction?
a. "I know to take my temperature if I get chills again like in the hospital."
b. "I won't exert myself around the house until I see the doctor."
c. "The nurse said to take more insulin when I start to eat more."*
d. "The social worker mentioned a support group. Maybe I should call about it."

† Adapted from *Review Questions for NCLEX–RN* (7th ed., pp. 7–8) by Sandra F. Smith, RN, MS. Copyright 1995 by National Nursing Review with permission.

MULTIPLE-RESPONSE

In multiple-response items several options may be correct, and students choose the best combination of responses. Principles for writing multiple-response items are the same as for multiple-choice. Additional suggestions include:

1. *The combination of alternatives should be plausible;* do not group options randomly, but instead consider how they might be logically combined.

2. *Use the alternatives a similar number of times in the combinations.* If one of the alternatives is in every combination, a clue is provided as to its correctness. Similarly, limited use of an option may provide a clue to the correct combination of responses. After grouping responses, count each letter to be sure that it is used a similar number of times across combinations of responses and that no letter is included in every combination.

3. *The responses should be listed in a logical order,* for instance, alphabetically or sequentially, for ease in reviewing.

A sample item follows:

Causes of cataracts include:
1. aging.
2. arteriosclerosis.
3. hemorrhage.
4. iritis.
5. steroid therapy.

a. 1, 2
b. 1, 5*
c. 2, 4
d. 1, 3, 4
e. 2, 3, 5

SUMMARY

The chapter described the development of multiple-choice and multiple-response items. Multiple-choice questions, with one correct or best answer, are used widely in nursing and other fields. This format of test item includes an incomplete statement or question, followed by a list of options that complete the statement or answer the question. Multiple-response items are designed similarly, although more than one answer may be correct. Both of these formats of test items may be used for evaluating learning at the recall, comprehension, application, and analysis levels, making them adaptable for a wide range of content and learning outcomes.

Multiple-choice items are important for testing application of nursing knowledge in simulated clinical situations and analytical thinking. Because of their versatility, they may be integrated easily within most testing situations.

There are three parts in a multiple-choice item, each with its own set of principles for development: (a) stem, (b) answer, and (c) distracters. The stem is the lead-in phrase in the form of a question or incomplete statement that relies on the alternatives for completion. Following the stem is a list of alternatives, options for the learner to consider and choose from. These alternatives are of two types: the answer, which is the correct or best alternative to answer the question or complete the statement, and distracters, which are the incorrect alternatives. Plausible distracters *distract* students who are unsure of the correct answer. Suggestions for writing each of these parts were presented in the chapter and were accompanied by sample items.

As students progress through a nursing program, they develop abilities to assess clients with varied needs and health problems, analyze data and derive multiple nursing diagnoses, set realistic goals for care considering the demands within the health care system, critique nursing interventions and select appropriate ones, and evaluate the effectiveness of care. Multiple-choice testing within the framework of the nursing process provides an opportunity to measure this learning. Items may be written about phases of the nursing process, decisions to be made in clinical situations and consequences of each, varying judgments possible in a situation, and other questions which examine students' critical thinking ability as related to the situation described in the test item. This format of multiple-choice testing also provides experience for students in answering the types of questions encountered in the NCLEX–RN.

Ability to write multiple-choice items is an important skill for the teacher to develop. This is a situation in which "practice makes perfect." After writing an item, have colleagues read it and make suggestions for revision. Try out questions with students and maintain a file of items for use in constructing tests. While this format is often time-consuming to develop, multiple-choice items provide an important means of evaluating learning in nursing.

REFERENCES

Ashley, J., & O'Neil, J. (1994). Study groups: Are they effective in preparing students for NCLEX–RN? *Journal of Nursing Education, 33,* 357–364.

Beare, P. G. (1995). NCLEX–RN update: Helping your students prepare. *Nurse Educator, 20*(3), 33–36.

Bloom, B. S., Englehart, M. D., Furst, E. J., Hill, W. H., & Krathwohl, D. R. (1956). *Taxonomy of educational objectives: The classification of educational goals. Handbook I: Cognitive domain.* New York: David McKay.

Bott, P. A. (1996). *Testing and assessment in occupational and technical education.* Boston: Allyn and Bacon.

Chenevey, B. (1988). Constructing multiple-choice examinations: Item writing. *Journal of Continuing Education in Nursing, 19,* 201–204.

Chornick, N. L., & Yocom, C. J. (1995). NCLEX job analysis study: Questionnaire development. *Journal of Nursing Education, 34,* 101–105.

Dell, M. S., & Valine, W. J. (1990). Explaining differences in NCLEX–RN scores with certain cognitive and non-cognitive factors for new baccalaureate nurse graduates. *Journal of Nursing Education, 29,* 158–162.

Eason, F., & Woolard, S. (1991). Report cards: A preparation strategy for NCLEX–RN. *Nurse Educator, 16*(1), 26–29.

Ebel, R. L., & Frisbie, D. A. (1991). *Essentials of educational measurement* (5th ed.). Englewood Cliffs, NJ: Prentice Hall.

Foti, I., & DeYoung, S. (1991). Predicting success on the National Council Licensing Examination-Registered Nurse: Another piece of the puzzle. *Journal of Professional Nursing, 7,* 99–104.

Gaberson, K. B. (1996). Test design: Putting all the pieces together. *Nurse Educator, 21*(4), 28–33.

Gronlund, N. E., & Linn, R. L. (1990). *Measurement and evaluation in teaching* (6th ed.). New York: Macmillan.

Horns, P. N., O'Sullivan, P., & Goodman, R. (1991). The use of progressive indicators as predictors of NCLEX–RN success and performance of BSN graduates. *Journal of Nursing Education, 30,* 9–14.

Hussey, C., Wolahan, C., & Wieczorek, R. (1991). Enrichment education: Key to NCLEX success. *Nursing & Health Care, 12,* 234–239.

Jenks, J., Selekman, J., Bross, T., & Paquet, M. (1989). Success in NCLEX–RN: Identifying predictors and optimal timing for intervention. *Journal of Nursing Education, 28,* 112–118.

Krupa, K. C., Quick, M. M., & Whitley, T. W. (1988). The effectiveness of nursing grades in predicting performance on the NCLEX–RN. *Journal of Professional Nursing, 4,* 294–298.

Kubiszyn, T., & Borich, G. (1993). *Educational testing and measurement* (4th ed.). New York: Harper Collins.

Lengacher, C. A., & Keller, R. (1990). Academic predictors of success on the NCLEX–RN examination for associate degree nursing students. *Journal of Nursing Education, 29,* 163–169.

McKinney, J., Small, S., O'Dell, N., & Coonrod, B. A. (1988). Identification of predictors of success for the NCLEX and students at risk for NCLEX failure in a baccalaureate nursing program. *Journal of Professional Nursing, 4,* 55–59.

Mills, A. C., Sampel, M. E., Pohlman, V. C., & Becker, A. M. (1992). The odds for success on NCLEX–RN by nurse candidates from a four-year baccalaureate nursing program. *Journal of Nursing Education, 31,* 403–408.

National Council of State Boards of Nursing. (1994). *NCLEX: Using CAT.* Chicago: Author.

National Council of State Boards of Nursing. (1995a). *Test plan for the National Council Licensure Examination for Registered Nurses.* Chicago: Author.

National Council of State Boards of Nursing. (1995b). *The NCLEX process.* Chicago: Author.

National Council of State Boards of Nursing. (1996). *Candidate information: NCLEX.* Chicago: Author.

Nitko, A. J. (1996). *Educational assessment of students* (2nd ed.). Englewood Cliffs, NJ: Prentice Hall.

Payne, M., & Duffey, M. (1986). An investigation of predictability of NCLEX–RN scores of BSN graduates using academic predictors. *Journal of Professional Nursing, 2,* 326–332.

Reilly, D. E., & Oermann, M. H. (1990). *Behavioral objectives: Evaluation in nursing* (3rd ed.). New York: National League for Nursing.

Smith, S. F. (1995). *Review questions for NCLEX–RN.* Los Altos, CA: National Nursing Review.

Yang, J. C., Glick, O, J., & McClelland, E. (1987). Academic correlates of baccalaureate graduate performance on NCLEX–RN. *Journal of Professional Nursing, 3,* 298–306.

6

Essay Test Items and Evaluation of Written Assignments

A n essay item is one in which the student develops an answer to a question, rather than choosing a correct response as was the case for many of the objective-type items described in the preceding chapters. Both essay tests and written assignments use writing as the medium of expressing the answer, although with essay items the focus of evaluation is the content of the answer rather than writing ability itself. Essay items and evaluation of written assignments are described in this chapter.

ESSAY ITEM

In an essay test, students construct responses to items based on their understanding of the content. With this type of test item, varied answers may be possible depending on the concepts selected by the student for discussion and the way in which they are presented. Essay items provide an opportunity for students to select content to discuss, present ideas in their own words, and develop an original and creative response to a question. This freedom of response makes essay items particularly useful for complex learning outcomes. Higher level responses, however, are more difficult to score than answers reflecting recall of facts. Although some essay items are developed around recall of facts and specific information, they are more appropriate for higher levels of learning. Gronlund and Linn (1990) recommended that essay items be used primarily for learning outcomes not able to be measured adequately through objective testing.

Although essay items use writing as the medium for expression, the intent is to evaluate student understanding of specific content, rather than to judge writing ability in and of itself. Other types of assignments are better suited to evaluating the ability of students to write effectively; these will be described later in the chapter. Low-level essay items are similar to short-answer and expect precise responses, for example, "Describe three signs of increased intracranial pressure in children under 2 years old." Broader and higher level essay items, however, do not limit responses in this way and differ clearly from short-answer items, such as "Defend the statement 'Access to health care is a right.'"

Essay items may be written to evaluate a wide range of learning outcomes. These include the following:

- comparing, such as comparing the side effects of two different medications;
- outlining steps to take and protocols to follow;
- explaining and summarizing in one's own words a situation or statement;
- discussing topics;
- applying concepts and principles to a situation and explaining their relevancy to it;
- analyzing client data and clinical situations through use of relevant concepts and theories;
- critiquing different interventions and nursing management;
- developing plans and proposals drawing upon multiple sources of information;
- analyzing health care and nursing trends;
- arriving at decisions about issues and actions to take accompanied by a rationale;
- analyzing ethical issues, possible decisions, and their consequences; and
- developing arguments for and against a particular position or decision.

As with other types of test items, the objective or outcome to be evaluated provides the framework for developing the essay item. From the objective, the teacher develops a clear and specific question to elicit information about student achievement in terms of the behavior and content specified in the objective. If the outcome to be evaluated specifies application of concepts to clinical practice, then the essay item should examine ability to apply knowledge to a client situation. Bott (1996) emphasized the need for clear questions that call for specific answers, not items that ask students to write all they know about a topic.

Reliability of Essay Tests and Issues in Scoring Responses

Although essay items are valuable for examining ability to select, organize, and present ideas, and they provide an opportunity for creativity and originality in responding, they are limited by low reliability and other issues associated with their scoring. These issues include:

1. *Limited ability to sample course content*: Essay items by their nature do not provide an efficient means of sampling course content in comparison with objective-type items. Bott (1996) suggested that essay tests have low reliability because of the "narrow sampling of the subject area" and issues in scoring.

2. *Teacher unreliability in scoring*: Hopkins, Stanley, and Hopkins (1990) identified the lack of consistency in evaluating essay responses among competent raters as a major limitation. Research in this area suggests that teachers are not consistent in their evaluations of answers to essay questions. Some teachers are more lenient than others, regardless of the criteria established for the evaluation and grading process. Teachers also vary in how they distribute the grades; some spread scores more widely than others, even if the scores cluster around an average score (Hopkins et al., 1990). Less restrictive essay items allowing for freedom and creativity in responding have even lower rater reliability than more restricted ones. When the essay item is highly focused and structured, such as "List three side effects of bronchodilators," there is greater reliability in scoring. Questions asking students to analyze, defend, judge, evaluate, critique, and develop products, however, are less reliable in terms of scoring the response. This unreliability in scoring even occurs when essays are reread by the same teacher (Hopkins et al., 1990, p. 202).

3. *Item-to-item carryover effect*: Hopkins et al. (1990) described another issue in evaluating essay questions as item-to-item carryover effect. In this situation, the teacher carries an impression of the quality of response from one item to the next. If the student answers one item well, the teacher may be influenced to score subsequent responses at a similarly high level; the same situation may occur with a poor response. The impression of the student is thus carried from one item to the next. For this reason, it is best to read all students' responses to one question before evaluating the next one.

4. *Test-to-test carryover effect*: A similar issue may occur if the teacher's impression of the student carries over from one test to the next. Once again, essay tests should be anonymous to avoid this influence on the evaluation.

5. *Halo effect*: In evaluating essay questions there may be a tendency to be influenced by a general impression of the student, a feeling about the

student that is either positive or negative, or other biases that may influence the teacher's judgment of the quality of the answers. For instance, the teacher may hold favorable opinions about the student in general, like the student, and believe the learner has made significant improvement in the course, which, in turn, might influence the scoring of responses. For this reason, essay tests should be rated anonymously.

6. *Effect of writing ability*: It is difficult to evaluate student responses based on content alone, even with clear and specific scoring guidelines. The teacher's rating is often influenced by sentence structure, grammar, spelling, punctuation, and overall writing ability. Bracht and Hopkins (1968) also reported that the length of the response influenced the rating, with longer answers receiving higher scores regardless of the content. Ebel and Frisbie (1991) believe that some students concentrate on "form rather than on content," presenting simple ideas elegantly as a way of diverting the teacher's attention away from a lack of knowledge (p. 190). The teacher, therefore, needs to evaluate the *content* of the learner's response and not be influenced by the writing style, unless this is incorporated as part of the scoring protocol.

7. *Order of grading effect*: The order in which essay tests are read and scored influences the evaluation. Essay tests read early tend to be scored higher than those read near the end. As such, teachers should read papers in random order and read each response twice before computing a score.

8. *Usability*: One other issue relates to the usability of essay items in terms of time for students to answer and for teachers to score. This becomes a pressing issue for teachers responsible for large numbers of students; in planning for essay tests, consideration should be given to the time required for correcting responses.

9. *Student choice of essay items*: Some essay tests allow students to choose a subset of questions to answer. This is often done because of limited time for testing and to provide options for students. Wainer, Wang, and Thissen (1994) cautioned, however, that the questions answered may not be comparable; a score of 10, for instance, on one item may not be comparable to this same score on a second, more difficult item. Often the items on an essay test are not of equal difficulty (Wainer & Thissen, 1994). Similarly, when students select different items to answer, their tests may not be comparable. If the items on the essay test assess important learning outcomes, then all students should answer all of them (Nitko, 1996, p. 169).

Restricted-Response Essay Items

There are two different types of essay items: restricted- and extended-response. Although the notion of freedom of response is inherent in essay items, there are varying degrees of this freedom in responding to the items. At one end of the continuum is the restricted-response item, in which a few sentences are required as indicated in the item. At the other end is the extended-response item, in which students have complete freedom of response, often requiring extensive writing. Responses to essay items fall typically between these two extremes.

In a restricted-response item, the teacher limits the student's answer by indicating the content to be presented and frequently the amount of discussion allowed, for instance, limiting the response to one paragraph or page. With this type of essay item, the way in which the student responds is structured by the teacher. A restricted-response item may be developed by posing a specific problem to be addressed and limiting the answer to this problem (Kubiszyn & Borich, 1993, p. 107). Specific material, such as patient data, description of a clinical situation, research findings, description of issues associated with clinical practice, and extracts from the literature, to cite a few examples, may be included with the essay item. Students are asked to read, analyze, and interpret this accompanying material, then answer questions about it or complete other tasks based on it (Nitko, 1996). Nitko (1996) defined these essay items as interpretive exercises or context-dependent tasks.

Examples of restricted-response items follow:

- Define "patient-focused care." Limit your definition to one paragraph.
- Select one environmental health problem and describe its potential effects on the community. Do not use an example presented in class. Limit your discussion to one page.
- Compare metabolic and respiratory acidosis. Include the following in your response: definitions, precipitating factors, clinical manifestations, diagnostic tests, and interventions.
- Mr. S is 76 years old and 1-day postoperative following a femoral popliteal bypass graft. Name two complications Mr. S could experience at this time and discuss why they are potential problems. List four nursing interventions for Mr. S during the initial recovery period and supporting rationale for each.
- Describe five physiological changes associated with the aging process.

Along a similar line, Takata (1994) proposed the guided essay examination. With this response format, students are given a basic outline to follow in responding to the essay question. The outline includes spaces to write an introduction, five topic statements, related subtopic state-

Describe how each family theoretical perspective would be used in providing nursing care for a family with a chronically ill child: structural –functional, systems, developmental, ecological, and stress. Which theoretical perspective would be most appropriate, if any, for this family? Why?

1. Introduction (introduction to family theories and their use in nursing)

2. Topic #1
    Subtopic A and related discussion
    Subtopic B and related discussion
    Subtopic C and related discussion

3. Topic #2
    Subtopic A and related discussion
    Subtopic B and related discussion
    Subtopic C and related discussion

4. Other topic (each with subtopic, related discussion, and space for answers)

5. Conclusions

Figure 6.1 Sample guided essay item.

ments with discussion, and a conclusion. Takata emphasizes that the outline, which accompanies the essay item and includes spaces for responding, assists students in organizing their ideas more clearly, restricts their responses, and facilitates grading. Figure 6.1 provides an example of an essay item and outline for answering, following Takata's (1994) model.

Extended-Response Essay Items

Extended-response essay items are less restrictive, and as such provide an opportunity for students to choose concepts for responding, organize ideas in their own ways, arrive at judgments about the content, and demonstrate ability to communicate ideas effectively in writing. With these items, the teacher may evaluate the students' ability to develop their own ideas and express them creatively, integrate learning from multiple sources in responding, and evaluate the ideas of others based on predetermined criteria. Since responses are not restricted by the teacher, evaluation is more difficult. This difficulty, however, is balanced by students being able to express their own ideas in response to an item. As such, essay questions provide a means of evaluating more complex learning that is not possible with objective-type items. The teacher may decide to allow students to respond to these items out of class.

Sample items include:

- Select an article describing a nursing research study. Critique the study, specifying the criteria used. Based on your evaluation, describe whether or not the research is of value to nursing practice.
- In the clinic you note that patients who are uninsured receive fewer diagnostic examinations and less comprehensive care than patients with similar health problems who are insured. Analyze these differences in care and related issues.
- Develop a plan for saving costs in the wound clinic.
- You receive a call in the allergy clinic from Mrs. J who describes her son's problems as "having stomach pains" and "acting out in school." She asks you if these problems may be due to his allergies. How would you respond to this mother? How would you manage this call? Include a rationale for your response.
- You are caring for a child diagnosed recently with acute lymphocytic leukemia who lives with his parents and two teenage sisters. Describe how the family health and illness cycle would provide a framework for assessing this family and planning care.

Writing Essay Test Items

Suggestions for developing essay items include:

1. *Develop items to measure the learning outcomes with responses that require grasp of essential content.* Avoid items that may be answered by merely summarizing the readings and class discussions without thinking about the content and applying it to new situations. Evaluating students' recall of facts and specific information may be accomplished more easily through objective testing than essay.

2. *Phrase items clearly.* The item should direct learners in their responses and should not be ambiguous. Table 6.1 provides sample stems for essay questions based on varied types of learning outcomes. Framing the item to make it as specific as possible is accomplished more easily with restricted response items. With extended response items, directions as to the type of response intended may be provided without limiting the student's own thinking about the answer. In example 1 (p. 101), there is minimal guidance as to how to respond; the revised version, however, directs students more clearly as to the intended response without limiting their freedom of expression and originality.

Table 6.1 Sample Stems for Essay Items

Comparing
Compare the side effects of . . . methods for . . . interventions for . . .
Describe similarities and differences between . . .
What do . . . have in common?
Group these medications . . . signs and symptoms . . .

Outlining Steps
Describe the process for . . . procedure for . . . protocol to follow
for . . .
List steps in order for . . .

Explaining and Summarizing
Explain the importance of . . . relevance of . . .
Identify and discuss . . .
Explain the patient's responses within the framework of . . .
Provide a rationale for . . .
Discuss the most significant points.
Summarize the relevant data.
What are the major causes of . . . reasons for . . . problems
associated with . . .
Describe the potential effects of . . . possible responses to . . .
problems which might result from . . .

Applying Concepts and Theories to a Situation
Analyze the situation using . . . theory/framework.
Using the theory of . . . , explain the client's/family's responses.
Identify and discuss . . . using relevant concepts and theories.
Discuss actions to take in this situation and theoretical basis.
Describe a situation that demonstrates the concept of . . . principle
of . . . theory of . . .

Analyzing
Discuss the significance of . . .
Identify relevant and irrelevant data with supporting rationale.
Identify and describe additional data needed for decision making.
Describe competing nursing diagnoses with rationale.
What hypotheses may be made?
Compare nursing interventions drawing upon research.
Describe multiple nursing interventions for this client with
supporting rationale.
Provide a rationale for...

(continued)

Table 6.1 *(cont.)*

Critique the nurse's responses to this client.
Describe errors in assumptions made about . . . errors in
    reasoning . . .
Analyze the situation and describe alternate actions possible.
Identify all possible decisions, consequences of each, your
    decision, and supporting rationale.

Developing Plans and Proposals
Develop a plan for . . . discharge plan . . . teaching plan . . .
Develop a proposal for . . . protocol for . . .
Based on the theory of . . . , develop a plan for . . . proposal for . . .
Develop a new approach for . . . method for . . .
Design multiple interventions for . . .
Write a research proposal.
Write an article about . . .
Write a report on . . .

Analyzing Trends and Issues
Identify one significant trend / issue in health care and describe
    implications for nursing practice.
Analyze this issue and implications for . . .
In light of these trends, what changes would you propose?
Critique the nurse's / physician's / client's decisions in this
    situation. What other approaches are possible? Why?
Analyze the ethical issue facing the nurse. Compare multiple
    decisions possible and consequences of each. Describe the
    decision you would make and why.
Identify issues for this client / family / community and strategies
    for resolving them.

Stating Positions
What would you do and why?
Identify your position about . . . and defend it.
Develop an argument for . . . and against . . .
Develop a rationale for . . .
Do you support this position? Why or why not?
Do you agree or disagree with . . . Include a rationale.
Specify the alternative actions possible. Which of these
    alternatives would be most appropriate and why? What
    would you do and why?

Example 1: Evaluate an article describing a nursing research study. *Revised version*: Select an article describing a nursing research study. Critique the study, specifying the criteria you used to evaluate it. Based on your evaluation, describe whether or not the research is of value to nursing practice.

3. Ebel and Frisbie (1991) recommended *including a larger number of specific items that may be answered briefly* rather than a few broad items. This strategy enables the teacher to sample the content domain more easily. It needs to be balanced, however, with the desire to include extended response questions, which allow for greater freedom in responding. Kubiszyn and Borich (1993) proposed that using more restricted response items improves scoring reliability.

4. *Prepare students for essay tests* by asking thought-provoking questions in class; engaging students in critical discussions about the content; and teaching students how to apply concepts and theories to situations, compare approaches, arrive at decisions and judgments about clients and issues, and organize ideas effectively. Practice with selecting concepts, presenting ideas logically, and using creativity in responding benefits students in completing essay items in a testing situation. This practice may be through class and clinical discussions, written assignments, and small group activities. For students lacking experience with essay tests, sample items may be used for formative purposes, providing feedback to students about the adequacy of their responses.

5. *Students should be told about apportioning their time*, allowing sufficient time to answer each essay item. In writing a series of essay items, consider carefully the time needed for students to answer them and inform students of the estimated time before they begin the examination. In this way, students may gauge their time appropriately.

6. For essay items dealing with analysis of issues, *students should provide a sound rationale for the position they take*. The rationale, rather than the actual position taken by the student, serves as the basis for evaluation.

7. *Avoid the use of optional items and student choice of items to answer*. As indicated previously, this results in different subsets of tests that may not be comparable.

8. *In the process of developing the item, write an ideal answer to it.* This should be done while drafting the item to determine if it is appropriate, clearly stated, and reasonable to answer in the allotted time frame. If possible, have a colleague review the item and explain how he or she would respond to it. Colleagues may be asked to judge the appropriateness of the question, breadth of coverage, difficulty level, and adequacy of the model answer (Hopkins et al., 1990, p. 216). Save this ideal answer for use later in scoring students' responses.

Scoring Essay Items

There are two methods of scoring essay items: holistic, also referred to as global impression, and analytical. The holistic method involves evaluating and assigning a score to the answer based on the overall quality of the response (Ebel & Frisbie, 1991, p. 195). In a norm-referenced system, each student's answer is compared to the responses of others in the group, a relative standard. To score essay questions using this system, the teacher reads quickly the answers to each question to gain a sense of how students responded overall, then rereads the answers and scores them. Papers may be placed in a number of piles reflecting degrees of quality, with each pile of papers receiving a particular score or grade. In a criterion-referenced approach, the student's answer is compared with an absolute standard, such as sample answers representing different degrees of quality (Ebel & Frisbie, 1991, p. 195). With this system, the teacher decides in advance characteristics of the answers expected for each possible score. For instance, a score of 3 might require all main points to be discussed with relevant concepts or theories cited as support. For a score of 2, 50% of the main points would be cited with relevant support, or all of the main points included but without discussion of the relevant theoretical base. A similar protocol would be developed for other possible scores.

In the analytical method of scoring, the teacher identifies the elements required in an ideal response. Each of these elements, which must be included in the answer, are evaluated and scored separately. Students accumulate points, therefore, based on the inclusion of these elements, not their responses overall. The analytical method of scoring is criterion-based. Ebel and Frisbie (1991) suggested that this method is well suited for essay items that yield detailed, structured answers (p. 196).

SUGGESTIONS FOR SCORING

1. *Identify the method of scoring* to be used prior to the testing situation and inform students of it.

2. *Specify in advance an ideal answer.* In constructing this ideal answer, review readings, classroom discussions of the content, and other instructional activities completed by students. Identify elements required in the answer and assign points to them if using the analytical method of scoring,

3. *In evaluating essay responses, consider the following criteria*:

- *Content.* Is relevant content included? Is it accurate? Are significant concepts and theories presented? Are hypotheses, conclusions, and decisions supported?

- *Organization.* Is the answer organized logically? Is there a logical sequence of ideas presented? Is the answer comprehensive?
- *Process.* Was the process used to arrive at solutions, actions, approaches, decisions, conclusions, and so forth adequate? Were consequences considered of varied decisions? Was the proper analysis carried out? Was a sound rationale provided? Did the student develop new ways of conceptualizing the problem? Solutions? (Kubiszyn & Borich, 1993).

4. *Read a random sample of papers* to get a sense of how students approached the items and notion of the overall quality of the answers.

5. *Score all the answers to one item at a time.* For example, read and score all of the students' answers to the first item before proceeding to the second item. This procedure enables the teacher to compare responses to an item across students, resulting in more accurate and fairer scoring, and saves time by requiring the teacher to keep in mind only one ideal answer at a time (Hopkins et al., 1990).

6. *Read each answer twice before scoring.* In the first reading, note omissions of major points from the ideal answer, errors in content, problems with organization, and problems with the process used for responding. Record corrections on the student's paper. After reading through all the answers to the question, begin the second reading for scoring purposes.

7. *Read papers in random order.*

8. *Use the same scoring system* for all student papers.

9. *Essay answers should be read anonymously.* Develop a system for implementing this in the nursing program, for instance, by asking students to choose a code number.

10. *Cover the scores of the previous answers* to avoid being biased about the student's ability.

11. If possible, *have a colleague read and score the answers to improve reliability.* A sample of answers might be independently scored rather than the complete set of student tests. For significant decisions, two or more independent ratings should be obtained (Gronlund & Linn, 1990, p. 226).

12. *Adopt a policy* as to the influence of sentence structure, spelling, punctuation, grammar, neatness, and writing style in general on the scoring, and inform students of this policy in advance of the test. Extended-response items developed to measure complex learning outcomes may be completed as out-of-class assignments; this provides more opportunity for producing well written responses.

WRITTEN ASSIGNMENTS

Written assignments, a predominant evaluation strategy used in nursing, serve two purposes: (a) to evaluate students' knowledge of content and (b) to evaluate their writing ability. In contrast to essay tests, which provide a means of judging mastery of content, written assignments enable the teacher to also evaluate ability to present, organize, and express ideas effectively in writing. Through papers and other written assignments, students develop an understanding of the content they are writing about and improve ability to communicate their ideas in writing. Allen, Bowers, and Diekelmann (1989) acknowledged the interrelationship between writing and thinking. Writing skills are enhanced through development of thinking skills, and thinking in turn is improved through writing exercises (p. 7).

McCarthy and Bowers (1994) described a writing-to-learn program that sequences written assignments across the nursing curriculum. These assignments begin with short, focused papers in which students summarize, in a few sentences, key points from lectures and readings, promoting a better understanding of how facts are selected and organized. This leads to other written assignments of varying lengths throughout the curriculum; faculty provide feedback on students' thinking and writing through drafts and rewrites of the papers. Benefits of critiquing written work, both by the student and teacher, were reported by Goldenberg (1994). Small-group critique of participants' writing also is appropriate, particularly for formative purposes. Writing papers collectively and evaluating the writing of others provides feedback among students and assists them in refining their thinking about the content and writing skills.

A common feature of writing assignments is submitting drafts of writing. "Through the student's interaction with his/her written work, each new draft pushes the student toward a better understanding of the content" (Allen et al., 1989, p. 7). In this way, writing assignments serve to teach content as well as improve writing. Drafts of written assignments are essential to foster development of writing skill. Short written assignments requiring multiple drafts that are critiqued by faculty in terms of accuracy of content, selection of concepts to present, development of ideas, organization of thoughts, and writing skills such as sentence structure, punctuation, and spelling serve to foster improvement of writing ability. The importance of learning to write effectively in nursing can not be underestimated. Poor writing style may prevent the nurse from sharing a great idea (Barnum, 1995).

There are many types of writing assignments appropriate for evaluation in nursing. Some of these assignments provide information on student achievement in terms of content but not necessarily writing skill, for example, nursing care plans and teaching plans, typically structured assignments involving short sentences and phrases with minimal opportunity for freedom of expression, originality, and creativity. Other assignments, however, provide data for judging acquisition of knowledge and content mastery as well as writing ability. Examples of written assignments include:

- Short in-class assignments in which students write down their thoughts about the content presented in class. These assignments may be reviewed by faculty, students, or both; papers also may be exchanged among students for peer review and discussion.
- Group writing assignments in class and clinical practice.
- Free writing assignments which are continuous and rapid writing with the goal of getting one's ideas on paper without concern about writing style and grammar (Bradley-Springer, 1993).
- Papers involving the analysis of concepts or issues (Lashley & Wittstadt, 1993).
- Term papers.
- Research papers and development of research proposals.
- Journal writing, recommended as one means of improving reading and writing skills as well as facilitating analysis and synthesis (Heinrich, 1992; Mann, 1996).
- Writing responses to editorials and articles in nursing (Berg & Serenko, 1993).
- Writing for publication (Davidhizar, 1993).

Evaluating Written Assignments

Whereas the evaluation of essay answers focuses predominantly on the quality of the content, in the case of written assignments the teacher has an opportunity to judge writing ability. Suggestions for developing and scoring essay items are also applicable to written assignments. Other considerations for evaluating written assignments include:

1. *Relate the assignments to the learning outcomes of the course.* Consider the number of written assignments to be completed by students, including drafts of papers. How many teaching plans, concept papers, research proposals, free writing exercises, one-page papers, and so forth are needed to meet the goals of the course?

2. *Avoid assignments that require only summarizing the literature* and sub-

stance of class discussions, unless this is the intended purpose of the assignment. Otherwise, students merely report on their readings, often without thinking about the content and how it relates to varied clinical situations. If a review of the literature is the outcome intended, have students read these articles critically and synthesize them as part of the written assignment, and not merely report on each article.

3. *Include clear directions about the purpose and format of the written assignment.* "What may seem a clear writing assignment to you [the teacher] may not be to students" (Mann, 1996, p. 35).

4. *Present the criteria for evaluation to students* prior to their beginning the assignment. Include criteria related to writing style, such as development and presentation of ideas, sentence structure, punctuation, grammar, spelling, length of the paper, references, and others.

5. *Specify the number of drafts to be submitted, each with required due dates.* Provide feedback promptly on quality of the content and writing, including specific suggestions about revisions. These drafts are a significant component of written assignments because the intent is to improve thinking and writing through them. Drafts in most instances are used as a means of providing feedback to students, and should not be scored.

6. *Consider incorporating student self-critique, peer-critique, and group writing exercises* within the sequence of assignments on writing.

7. *Prepare students for written assignments* by incorporating learning activities in the course, completed both in and out of class, which provide practice in organizing and expressing ideas in writing.

8. For papers dealing with analysis of issues, *focus the evaluation and criteria on the rationale developed for the position taken,* rather than the actual position. This type of assignment is particularly appropriate as a group activity with critique of each other's work.

9. Principles for scoring written assignments are similar to those described for essay questions. *Develop a scoring system,* based on criteria related to quality of content and writing, and apply the system comparably across students. Papers should be read anonymously. Read them twice before scoring and in a random order for both readings. An average paper may appear of higher quality in terms of the criteria if it follows a poorly written one.

10. When possible, *provide for multiple independent ratings of papers.*

SUMMARY

This chapter presented important principles for developing and evaluating essay items and written assignments. In an essay test, students construct responses to items based on their understanding of the content. With this type of test item, varied answers may be possible depending on the concepts selected by the student for discussion and the way in which they are presented. Essay items provide an opportunity for students to select content to discuss, present ideas in their own words, and develop original and creative responses to items. This freedom of response makes essay items particularly useful for complex learning outcomes.

Although essay items use writing as the medium for expression, the intent is to evaluate student understanding of specific content, rather than judge writing ability in and of itself. Other types of assignments are better suited to evaluating the ability of students to write effectively.

There are two different types of essay items: restricted- and extended-response. In a restricted-response item, the teacher limits the student's answer by indicating the content to be presented and frequently the amount of discussion allowed, for instance, limiting the response to one paragraph or page. With this type of essay item, the way in which the student responds is structured by the teacher. In an extended-response item, students have complete freedom of response, often requiring extensive writing. Answers to essay items fall typically in between these two extremes.

Written assignments, a predominant evaluation strategy used in nursing, serve two purposes: to evaluate students' knowledge of content and their writing ability. In contrast to essay tests, which provide a means of judging mastery of content, written assignments also enable the teacher to evaluate ability to present, organize, and express ideas effectively in writing. Through papers and other written assignments, students develop an understanding of the content they are writing about and improve their ability to communicate their ideas in writing. Suggestions for developing and scoring essay items are also applicable to written assignments with the addition of criteria related to writing skill, such as development and presentation of ideas, sentence structure, punctuation, grammar, spelling, length of the paper, and references. Written assignments provide a means of judging complex and higher levels of learning, evaluating ability to communicate ideas effectively in writing, and an opportunity for originality and creativity in responding.

REFERENCES

Allen, D. G., Bowers, B., & Diekelmann, N. (1989). Writing to learn: A reconceptualization of thinking and writing in the nursing curriculum. *Journal of Nursing Education, 28*, 6–11.

Barnum, B. S. (1995). *Writing and getting published.* New York: Springer Publishing.

Berg, J., & Serenko, P. C. (1993). Teaching professional writing skills to the baccalaureate student. *Journal of Nursing Education, 32,* 329.

Bott, P. A. (1996). *Testing and assessment in occupational and technical education.* Boston: Allyn and Bacon.

Bracht, G. H., & Hopkins, K. D. (1968). *Comparative validities of objective tests.* (Research paper No. 20.) Boulder, CO: University of Colorado. (As cited in Hopkins, K. D., Stanley, J. C., & Hopkins, B. R. (1990). *Educational and psychological measurement and evaluation* (7th ed.). Englewood Cliffs, NJ: Prentice Hall.)

Bradley-Springer, L. (1993). Discovery of meaning through imagined experience, writing, and evaluation. *Nurse Educator, 18*(5), 5–10.

Davidhizar, R. (1993). Mentoring nursing students to write. *Journal of Nursing Education, 32,* 280–282.

Ebel, R. L., & Frisbie, D. A. (1991). *Essentials of educational measurement* (5th ed.). Englewood Cliffs, NJ: Prentice Hall.

Goldenberg, D. (1994). Critiquing as a method of evaluation in the classroom. *Nurse Educator, 19*(4), 18–22.

Gronlund, N. E., & Linn, R. L. (1990). *Measurement and evaluation in teaching* (6th ed.). New York: Macmillan.

Heinrich, K. T. (1992). The intimate dialogue: Journal writing by students. *Nurse Educator, 17*(6), 17–21.

Hopkins, K. D., Stanley, J. C., & Hopkins, B. R. (1990). *Educational and psychological measurement and evaluation* (7th ed.). Englewood Cliffs, NJ: Prentice Hall.

Kubiszyn, T., & Borich, G. (1993). *Educational testing and measurement* (4th ed.). New York: Harper Collins.

Lashley, M., & Wittstadt, R. (1993). Writing across the curriculum: An integrated curricular approach to developing critical thinking through writing. *Journal of Nursing Education, 32,* 422–424.

Mann, S. A. (1996). Respect: Improving student writing. *Nurse Educator, 21*(4), 34–36.

McCarthy, D. O., & Bowers, B. (1994). Implementation of writing-to-learn in a program of nursing. *Nurse Educator, 19*(3), 32–35.

Nitko, A. J. (1996). *Educational assessment of students* (2nd ed.). Englewood Cliffs, NJ: Prentice Hall.

Takata, S. R. (1994). The guided essay examination for sociology and other courses. *Teaching Sociology, 22,* 189–194.

Wainer, H., & Thissen, D. (1994). On examinee choice in educational testing. *Review of Educational Research, 64*(1), 159–195.

Wainer, H., Wang, X., & Thissen, D. (1994). *Journal of Educational Measurement, 31*(3), 183–199.

7

Evaluation of Problem Solving, Decision Making, and Critical Thinking: Context-Dependent Item Sets and Other Evaluation Strategies

I n preparing students to care for clients with complex health needs and to function within the changing health care system, teachers are faced with identifying essential content to teach within the nursing education program. Mastery of this knowledge alone, however, will not enable students to arrive at critical decisions about their patients. In addition to acquiring a knowledge base for practice, students and nurses alike need to develop cognitive skills for processing and analyzing information, comparing different approaches, weighing alternatives, and arriving at sound conclusions and decisions. These cognitive skills include, among others, problem solving, decision making, and critical thinking.

Although there are varied perspectives of each of these cognitive skills, broad generalizations are used in this chapter to provide a framework for presenting strategies for evaluating and testing these abilities. It is acknowledged that these processes are interrelated. One view is that critical thinking is the thought process that underlies problem solving and decision making (Oermann, 1997). Critical thinking enables the student to reframe the problem, remaining open to new perspectives (Case, 1994); consider different problems; evaluate alternate approaches possible; consider the consequences of each; and arrive at sound decisions after carefully weighing the evidence. Critical thinking skills are used throughout the problem-solving and decision-making processes. For the purpose of this chapter, however, these cognitive skills are considered separately to illustrate how test items and other evaluation strategies may be developed for them.

PROBLEM SOLVING

In the practice setting, students are faced continually with client and other problems to be solved. Some of these problems relate to managing client, family, and community health needs; others involve problems associated with one's role and work environment. Ability to solve client and setting-related problems is an essential skill to be developed and evaluated. Problem solving begins with recognizing and defining the problem, gathering data to clarify it further, developing solutions and evaluating their effectiveness. Knowledge about the problem and potential solutions, from a theoretical point of view, influences the problem-solving process. Students faced with client problems of which they lack understanding and a relevant knowledge base will be impeded in their thinking. This is an important point in both teaching and evaluating problem-solving ability; students need a knowledge base upon which to base their problem solving. Kintgen-Andrews (1991) suggested that understanding of the content is an important factor in problem solving.

Past experience with similar problems, either real problems in the clinical setting or hypothetical ones used in teaching, also influences skill in problem solving. Experience with similar problems gives the student a perspective of what to expect in the clinical situation, of typical problems the client may experience as well as solutions that are often effective. Benner (1984) reported that expert nurses and beginners, such as students, approached problems differently. Experts, because of their clinical experience, view the client situation as a whole and use their past experience with similar clients as a framework for approaching new problems.

Cognitive Development

Problem-solving skill is influenced in general by the student's level of cognitive development. Perry's (1970) theory of cognitive development suggests that students progress in their thinking through four stages:

- *Dualism:* In this first stage, students view knowledge and values as absolutes. In terms of problem solving, they look for one problem with accepted solutions often reflecting their readings and prior learning. At this stage, students are unable to consider the possibility of different problems and varied solutions to them.

- *Multiplicity:*In the second stage, students are willing to acknowledge that the problems may be different from the first ones identified, and varied solutions may be possible. They begin to accept the notion that multiple points of view are possible in a given situation. In this stage, learners are able to see shades of gray and multiple truths (Hursh, Haas, & Moore, 1983).
- *Relativism:*In the third stage of relativism, students possess the cognitive ability and willingness to evaluate different points of view. At this stage in their cognitive development, students have progressed in their thinking to the point that they can evaluate varying perspectives and approaches relative to one another.
- *Commitment in relativism:*Perry's final stage of cognitive development reflects a commitment to identify one's values and beliefs and act on them in practice.

Perry's theory provides a way of viewing the development of cognitive skills among nursing students. Skill in problem solving and other cognitive abilities may reflect the student's stage of cognitive development. Complexity of thinking and problem solving, acceptance of multiple perspectives, ability to deal with ambiguity, willingness to take risks, and commitment to act on one's values and beliefs occur at advanced stages of cognitive development (Reilly & Oermann, 1992, p. 220).

Well-Structured and Ill-Structured Problems

Nitko (1996) defined two types of problems students may be asked to solve: well-structured and ill-structured. Well-structured problems provide the information needed for problem solving, typically have one correct solution rather than multiple ones to consider, and in general are "clearly laid out" (p. 185). These are problems and solutions that the teacher may have presented in class and then asks students about in the evaluation. Well-structured problems provide practice in applying concepts and theories learned in class to hypothetical situations, but do not require extensive critical thinking skills.

In contrast, ill-structured problems reflect real-life problems and clinical situations faced by students. With these situations the problem may not be clear to the learner; different problems may be possible, given the data; or there may be an incomplete data set to determine the problem. Along a similar line, the student may identify the problem but be unsure of the approaches to take; multiple solutions also may be possible. Some evaluation strategies for problem solving address well-structured problems, assessing understanding of typical problems and solutions. Other evaluation methods assess ability to analyze situations to identify different problems possible given the data, identify additional data needed to decide on a particular problem, compare and evaluate multiple approaches, and arrive at an informed decision as to actions to take in the situation.

DECISION MAKING

The nurse continually makes decisions about client care—decisions about problems, solutions, alternate approaches that might be possible, and the best approach to use in a particular situation. Other decisions are needed for delivering care, managing the clinical environment, and carrying out other activities. As such, skill in decision making reflects another outcome of the nursing program.

In decision making, the learner arrives at a decision after considering a number of alternatives and weighing the consequences of each. The decision reflects a choice after considering these different possibilities. In making this choice, the student compares possible alternatives and the consequences of each, then arrives at a decision as to the best strategy or approach to use (Reilly & Oermann, 1992). There are three broad phases in decision making significant in designing the evaluation:(a) collection and analysis of information in the situation relevant to identifying the problem and making a decision, (b) consideration of different alternatives possible and consequences of each, and (c) arriving at a decision as to the best alternative for the situation.

CRITICAL THINKING

The importance of developing ability to think critically in nursing cannot be underestimated. The complexity of client, family, and community needs; amount of information the nurse needs to process in the practice setting; types of decisions required for care and supervising others in the delivery of care; and multiple ethical issues faced by the nurse all require the ability to think critically. Critical thinking is needed to make reasoned and informed judgments in the practice setting. Through critical thinking, the nurse is able to decide what to do in a given situation (Facione & Facione, 1996). Kataoka-Yahiro and Saylor (1994) defined critical thinking as reflective and reasoned thinking about nursing problems without one solution, focused on decisions about what to believe and do.

Critical thinking is disciplined, well-reasoned thinking based on intellectual standards such as "relevancy, accuracy, precision, clarity, depth, and breadth" (Paul, 1993, p. 20). There are eight elements of reasoning to be considered in the process of critical thinking:

1. Purpose the thinking is to serve,
2. Question, issue, or problem to be resolved,
3. Assumptions on which thinking is based,
4. Analysis of own point of view and those of others,
5. Data, information, and evidence on which to base reasoning,
6. Concepts and theories for use in thinking,
7. Inferences and conclusions possible given the data,
8. Implications and consequences of reasoning. (Foundation for Critical Thinking, 1994)

These elements of reasoning may be used as a framework for evaluating students' critical thinking in nursing. Sample questions the teacher might ask in assessing if students are considering these elements in their reasoning are presented in Table 7.1.

In the clinical setting, critical thinking enables the student to arrive at sound and rational decisions to carry out care of clients. Carrying out assessment; planning care; intervening with clients, families, and communities; and evaluating the effectiveness of interventions require critical thinking. In the assessment process, important cognitive skills include differentiating relevant from irrelevant data, identifying cues in the data and clustering them, planning additional data to collect prior to arriving at decisions as to the problem, and specifying patient problems and nursing diagnoses based on these data. Ability to generate competing diagnoses and evaluate each one is another important skill. Critical thinking also is reflected in ability to compare different approaches possible, considering the consequences of each, and arrive at a decision as to nursing measures and approaches to use in a particular situation (Oermann, 1997). Judgments about the quality and effectiveness of care are influenced by the learner's critical thinking skill. It is through critical thinking that the student begins to consider and evaluate multiple perspectives to care.

Students who demonstrate critical thinking ability:

- ask questions in class and clinical practice;
- are inquisitive and willing to search for answers;
- consider alternate ways of viewing information;
- offer different perspectives to problems and solutions;
- question current practices and express their own ideas about care;
- extend their thinking beyond the readings, class instruction, clinical activities, and other requirements; and
- are open-minded.

Table 7.1 Sample Questions for Evaluating Critical Thinking

Do students:

Purpose of critical thinking

State the purpose of their critical thinking?
State goals to be achieved as a result of their critical thinking?
Use this purpose and these goals to stay focused with their
thinking?
Have realistic and attainable goals?

Issue or problem to be resolved

Clarify the issue or problem to be resolved?
Divide issues and problems into manageable ones for resolution?
Ask probing questions to clarify the issue or problem further?
Focus on important and significant issues and problems?
Raise questions relevant to resolving the issue or problem?
Ask questions that are unbiased?
Recognize questions they are unable to answer and seek
information independently for answering them?

Assumptions on which thinking is based

Make assumptions that are clear? Reasonable? Consistent with
one another?
Question assumptions underlying their own thinking?

Analysis of own point of view and that of others

Keep in mind different points of view?
Realize that people approach situations, questions, issues, and
problems differently?
Consider multiple perspectives?
Have a broad point of view about issues and problems, rather
than a narrow perspective?
Recognize their own biases, values, and beliefs that influence
their thinking and how they see others' points of view?
Seek actively others' points of view?

Information and evidence on which to base reasoning

Collect sufficient data and evidence on which to base their
thinking?
Base their reasoning and points of view on relevant data and
evidence?
Search for information for and against their position and critically
analyze both sets of data?
Differentiate relevant and irrelevant information for the question,
issue, or problem at hand?
Avoid drawing conclusions beyond the information and evidence
available to support them?

(continued)

Table 7.1 *(cont.)*

Present clear and accurate data and evidence on which their thinking is based?

Concepts and theories for use in thinking
Apply relevant concepts and theories for understanding and analyzing the question, issue, or problem?
Avoid biases in presentation of ideas and thinking?
Recognize implications of words used in presenting ideas?
Avoid misuse of concepts and theories?

Inferences and conclusions
Make clear and precise inferences?
Clarify their conclusions and make their reasoning easy to follow?
Draw conclusions based on the evidence and reasons presented?
Draw conclusions that are consistent with one another?

Implications and consequences of reasoning
Identify a number of significant implications of their thinking?
Identify different courses of action and consequences of each?
Consider both positive and negative consequences?

Note. From *Critical Thinking Workshops.* (pp. 20–27), by Foundation for Critical Thinking, 1994, Santa Rose, CA: Author. Copyright 1994 by Foundation for Critical Thinking. Adapted with permission.

Case (1994) identified another important characteristic as willingness to evaluate and challenge, rather than accept. A questioning attitude permeates the critical thinking process in nursing and other fields. These characteristics of critical thinking are important so the strategies for evaluation provide information on the students' underlying thought processes, not only on the outcome and product of their thinking.

EVALUATION OF PROBLEM SOLVING, DECISION MAKING, AND CRITICAL THINKING

In assessing students' cognitive skills, the test items and evaluation methods need to meet two criteria. They should (a) introduce new information not encountered by students at an earlier point in the instruction and (b) provide data on the thought process used by students to arrive at an answer, rather than the answer alone. Context-dependent item sets may be used for this purpose. Other evaluation methods include: case method and study, discussion, debate, media clips, written assignments, and varied clinical evaluation methods that are presented in chapter 11. Lastly, standardized tests are available to measure general critical thinking ability, although these are not specific to critical thinking in nursing.

Writing Context-Dependent Item Sets

In evaluating higher level skills, the teacher as a basic principle needs to introduce new or novel material for analysis. Without the introduction of new material as part of the evaluation, students may have memorized from prior discussion or their readings how to problem solve and arrive at decisions for the situation at hand; they may recall the typical problem and solutions without thinking through other possibilities themselves. In nursing, this is frequently accomplished by developing clinical scenarios that present a novel situation for students to apply concepts and theories, problem solve, arrive at decisions, and in general engage in critical thinking. Nitko (1996) referred to these items as context-dependent item sets or interpretative exercises.

In a context-dependent item set, the teacher presents introductory material that students then analyze and answer questions about. The introductory material may be a description of a clinical situation, patient data, research findings, issues associated with clinical practice, and varied types of scenarios; students then read, analyze, and interpret this material and answer questions about it or complete other tasks. The introductory material also may include diagrams, photographs, graphs, charts, excerpts from reading materials, and media (Nitko, 1996, p. 177). One advantage of a context-dependent item set is the opportunity to present new information for student analysis geared toward clinical practice. In addition, the introductory material provides the same context for problem solving, decision making, and critical thinking for all students (Nitko, 1996).

Although one item may be developed around the introductory material, in most instances the teacher will plan a series of items related to the same content. Test items for evaluating the nursing process, described in chapter 5, may be developed in the form of context-dependent items with a series of questions about one clinical scenario. With objective-type items, however, the teacher is not able to assess the underlying thought process used by students in arriving at the answer; their choice of responses reflects instead the outcome of their thinking. For this reason, context-dependent item sets for evaluating higher-level cognitive skills typically involve open-ended questions, such as short-answer and essay.

Suggestions follow for writing context-dependent item sets. The examples in this chapter are designed for paper-and-pencil testing; however, the scenarios and other types of introductory material for analysis may be presented through multimedia, computer-assisted instruction, interactive video, and other types of technology.

1. If the intent is to evaluate students' skills in problem solving, decision making, and critical thinking, *the introductory material needs to provide sufficient*

information for analysis without directing the students' thinking in a particular direction. Draft the types of questions to be asked about the situation, then develop a scenario to provide essential information for analysis. If the scenario is designed around clinical practice, students may be asked to analyze data, identify patient problems, decide on nursing measures, evaluate outcomes of care, and examine ethical issues, among other tasks.

2. *The questions should focus on the underlying thought process used to arrive at an answer,* not the answer alone. In some situations, however, the goal may be to assess ability to apply principles or procedures learned in class without considering any original thinking about them. In these instances, well-structured problems with one correct answer and situations that are clearly laid out for students are appropriate.

3. *The introductory material should be geared to the students' level of understanding and experience.* Check carefully the terminology used, particularly with beginning students. The situation should be a reasonable length without extending students' reading time unnecessarily.

4. *Specify how the responses will be scored,* if they are restricted in some way, such as page length, and the criteria used for evaluation. Context-dependent items may be completed individually or in small groups, in class, as part of the clinical practice experience, or as out-of-class assignments. If group work is evaluated for summative purposes, students should have an opportunity to evaluate each other's participation. Figure 7.1 provides a sample form for this purpose.

5. Item sets focusing on assessment of problem-solving ability may ask students to complete the following tasks:
- identify the problem and alternate problems possible;
- develop questions for clarifying the problem further;
- identify assumptions made about the problem and solutions;
- identify additional data needed for decision making;
- differentiate relevant and irrelevant information in the situation (Nitko, 1996, p. 187);
- propose solutions, alternatives possible, advantages and disadvantages of each, and their choices;
- identify obstacles to solving a problem;
- relate information from different sources to the problem to be solved;
- work backwards from the desired outcome to develop a plan for solving the problem (Nitko, 1996, p. 189);
- evaluate the effectiveness of solutions and approaches to solving problems and the outcomes achieved.

Examples of item sets reflecting these tasks are provided in the boxes that follow.

Student's name _____

Group project _____

Date _____

Rate each of the behaviors listed below by circling the appropriate number. Complete a rating of each student in your group.

Behaviors	Rating				
	Poor				Excellent
Participates actively in group discussions	1	2	3	4	5
Offers new perspectives to group	1	2	3	4	5
Considers different points of view	1	2	3	4	5
Assists group members in recognizing biases and values that may influence discussions and decision making	1	2	3	4	5
Is enthusiastic about group work	1	2	3	4	5
Completes on time own share of work	1	2	3	4	5
Develops quality materials and products for group	1	2	3	4	5
Shares responsibilities of group work	1	2	3	4	5
Assists other group members with their responsibilities	1	2	3	4	5
Gathers resources for the group	1	2	3	4	5

Figure 7.1 Evaluation of individual participation in group work.

Mrs. B, a 36-year-old patient scheduled for a breast biopsy, has been crying on and off for the last 3 hours during her diagnostic testing. When the nurse attempts to talk to Mrs. B about her feelings, Mrs. B says, "Everything is fine. I'm just tired."

1. What is the problem in this situation that needs to be solved?
2. What assumptions about Mrs. B did you make in identifying this problem?
3. What additional information would you collect from Mrs. B and her health records before intervening? Why is this information important?

Mr. J received immunotherapy 10 minutes ago. He returns to the clinic stating he "feels funny and itches all over."

1. What questions should be asked and what observations should be made to identify Mr. J's problem?

Michael, your 8-year-old patient, had a closed head injury 4 weeks ago after falling off his bike. You visit him at home and find that he has weakness of his left leg. His mother reports that he is "getting his rest" and "sleeping a lot." Michael seems irritable during your visit. When you ask him how he is feeling, he tells you,"My head hurts where I hit it."The mother appears anxious, talking rapidly and changing position frequently.

1. List all possible problems in this situation. For each problem describe supporting assessment data.
2. What additional data are needed, if any, to decide on these problems? Provide a rationale for collecting this information.
3. What other assessment data would you collect at this time? Why is this information important to your decision making?

Mr. S is admitted with sharp chest pain during inspiration and shortness of breath. His PaO2 level is 75 and his oxygen saturation is 80%. The preliminary diagnosis is pulmonary embolism.

1. List potential nursing diagnoses with supporting rationale.
2. What additional data are needed to support or reject each diagnosis?

Mr. P has undergone a radical prostatectomy. His wife is a physician at the hospital. Following the surgery she asks you to bring his chart to the room.

1. What are two approaches you could use in this situation? Identify advantages and disadvantages of each.
2. What would you say to Mr. P's wife after her request? What is your reasoning for responding in this way?
3. What obstacles do you face in solving this problem?

The American Nurses Association (ANA) *Code for Nurses* states that "the nurse safeguards the client's right to privacy by judiciously protecting information of a confidential nature." Jenna, a 15-year-old, is seen by the nurse practitioner in the clinic for nausea. She is brought there by her mother. When the mother leaves the room, Jenna confides in the nurse practitioner that she is pregnant.

1. What are different options for the nurse practitioner at this time? Describe advantages and disadvantages of each.
2. How would you solve this dilemma? Include in your answer how you used the ANA *Code for Nurses* in your proposed solution.

You are working in a clinic in which many of the clients are drug users. They experience recurring wounds. You note that the nurse practitioners who see these patients use different wound treatments than the ET nurse. In a meeting the group decides to plan a research study to compare these treatments.

1. Design this research study, including the steps you would take and related time frame. You may add information to the situation described above to clarify the process you would use in designing the study.

Jane is a 1-month-old brought to the pediatrician's office for a well-baby checkup. You notice that she has not gained much weight over the last month. Jane's mother explains that Jane is "colicky" and "spits up a lot of her feeding." There is no evidence of projectile vomiting and other GI symptoms. Jane has a macular-type rash on her stomach, her temperature is normal, and she appears well hydrated.

1. Describe at least three different nursing interventions that could be used in this situation. Provide a rationale for each.
2. What would you do in this situation? Why is the approach you selected better than the others?
3. Specify outcome criteria for evaluating the effectiveness of the intervention you selected.
4. What information presented in this situation is irrelevant to your decision making? Why?

6. Context-dependent items may focus on actions to be taken in a situation. For this purpose, *describe briefly a critical event, then ask for actions to take*. For example:

Mrs. D's pulmonary capillary wedge pressure has been 14 mmHg. You take it and find it is 6 mmHg.

1. What would you do first? Why?

You are interviewing residents of a nursing home. When you enter your patient's room, you find him tied to the arms of his wheelchair.

1. What would you do? Why did you choose this action?

---

7. *For assessment of decision-making ability*, two approaches may be used with the item set. The introductory material (a) may present a situation up to the point of a decision, then ask students to make a decision or (b) may describe a situation and decision and ask whether they agree or disagree with it. For both of these approaches, students need to provide a rationale for their responses. An example of each of these types of decision-making items is provided in the boxes that follow.

Ms. J is your nurse manager on a busy surgery unit. She asks you to cover for her while she attends a meeting. You find out later that she left the hospital to run errands instead of attending the meeting.

1. Identify three alternate courses of action that could be taken in this situation.
2. Describe the possible consequences of each course of action.
3. What decision would you make? Why?

An asthmatic patient receiving immunotherapy calls to see if he should receive his injection today. He had been ill, but he returned to work yesterday. The nurse gathers the following information:The patient is afebrile and has a clear productive cough and mild headache. The nurse instructs the patient to come in for his injection.

1. Do you agree or disagree with the nurse's decision? Why or why not?

---

8. *Test items may be of any format*, although if the intent is to evaluate higher level cognitive skills, open-ended items provide the most effective way of assessing the underlying thought process used by students. If this is not essential, then other types of items, such as multiple-choice, are also appropriate.

9. *Context-dependent item sets also may be developed for assessing critical thinking skills*. Paul's (1993) elements of reasoning provide a framework for designing questions for this purpose. Suggestions follow for developing these questions.

Develop scenarios with problems to be solved, issues to be addressed, and questions to be answered

---

Ask students to:
- Identify the problems and issues to be solved and supporting rationale;
- Clarify the problems and issues further by raising careful and pointed questions;
- Describe how they would go about solving the problems, resolving the issues, and answering the questions;
- Identify multiple approaches for these problems and issues and consequences of each approach;
- Decide on the approach they would use and provide a rationale underlying their thinking;
- Examine how key concepts and ideas are used in analyses of situations; and
- Identify assumptions they made and how these influenced their thinking.

Develop a situation with different points of view as to the problem, issue, or approaches to use.

Ask students to:
- Articulate the different points of view and reasoning behind each one;
- Examine the data, information, and evidence on which these points of view are based;
- Evaluate the evidence used to support a particular position;
- Make inferences and draw conclusions that follow from the evidence and reasoning presented; and
- Compare varied decisions possible in a situation and outcomes.

Many of the examples of item sets presented earlier assess critical thinking skills within the context of problem solving and decision making. A few other examples follow:

Mr. E is a 68-year-old dialysis patient. He has been depressed lately and appears tired. He asks you if he can refuse further dialysis treatments.

1. How would you respond to Mr. E? Why is this an appropriate response?
2. What questions would you ask Mr. E?
3. What are issues to be resolved in this situation?

The *Social Policy Statement* indicates that nursing is "owned by society" (ANA, 1995, p. 2).

1. What is the reasoning behind this statement?
2. Describe another point of view and provide evidence to support it.

The following items are based on your readings:

Reading A   Reading B   Reading C

1. From these readings on financing health care, draw five conclusions supported by all three readings.
2. What is the most fundamental difference between Readings A and B in terms of rationing health care? Identify underlying assumptions of each of these positions.
3. What are the implications of these positions on rationing health care?

Discussion was held about the costs of maintaining the geriatric nurse practitioners at the long-term care facility. One board member suggested that nursing assistants would be able to meet many of the patient needs at lower cost. Her suggestion was based on prior experience at another nursing home in which there were no practitioners and patients still received adequate care.

1. What questions would you ask this board member?
2. What are issues, if any, with the suggestion?
3. How would you evaluate the credibility of the board member to make this suggestion?

After viewing the video clip, answer the following questions:

1. Do you think the nurse's response to the family was misleading? Why or why not?

The following item refers to these advertisements on HMOs.
Advertisement A   Advertisement B

1. Once a year employees of the hospital are able to change their health insurance. The above advertisements are for two new HMOs available to employees. Based on your readings, are either of these advertisements misleading? Why or why not?

A follow-up study of graduates of a nursing program found that 80% of the students who completed a course in critical care nursing worked as graduates in critical care.

1. Which of the following interpretations of this finding is most valid? Circle your response.
   a. Completing a critical care course as a student may be related to future practice in critical care.
   b. Graduates of the nursing program are more likely to practice in critical care than other nursing specialties.
   c. If you take a critical care course as a student, you will be prepared for employment in critical care.
   d. The more experience you gain as a student in critical care, the better prepared you will be as a graduate to practice in critical care.
   e. Working in critical care as a graduate requires a prior course in critical care as a student.
2. Provide a rationale for your answer.

Evaluation Strategies for Higher Level Cognitive Skills

Although context-dependent item sets provide one means of testing higher level cognitive skills, other evaluation methods are available for this purpose: case method and study, discussion, debate, media clips, short written assignments, standardized testing, and varied clinical evaluation methods presented in chapter 11. Many of the evaluation strategies described in this section of the chapter also may be used for clinical evaluation.

CASE METHOD AND CASE STUDY

Fuszard (1995) differentiated case method from case study. In case method, students analyze a problem under the direction of the teacher, reach consensus on the case, and then discuss the implications of their decisions (p. 81). With the *case method*, students are given a case for analysis, they review related literature, and as a group they solve problems inherent in the case. Following the analysis of the case, the teacher and students can review the theoretical issues involved in the case to promote application to future cases (Fuszard, 1995, p. 84).

Reilly and Oermann (1990, 1992) described three different case methods:

1. *Problem solving,* in which a situation was presented for students to identify problems and solutions through application of relevant concepts and theories;
2. *Decision making,* requiring one or more decisions as part of the analysis; and
3. *Critical incident,* in which students analyzed a critical event and identified actions to take.

Regardless of the perspective, case method provides an important strategy for evaluating ability to analyze a case, identify problems and solutions, compare alternate decisions possible, and arrive at conclusions about different aspects of the case. Case method is an effective strategy for small groups, providing a way for students to critique each others' thinking; gain other perspectives of the problem, solutions, and decisions possible; and learn how to arrive at a group consensus regarding decisions. Used as a small group activity, case method is more easily evaluated for formative purposes than summative.

A *case study* provides a hypothetical or real-life situation for students to analyze and arrive at varied decisions. Case studies are typically longer and more comprehensive than the introductory material presented with case method. As such, with case studies students are able to provide detailed and in-depth analyses and describe the evidence on which their conclusions are based. The reasoning used by students to identify questions, problems, and issues and think through their solutions may be evaluated through a case study by asking students to provide the rationale underlying their thinking. The case study method also provides an avenue for students to apply relevant concepts and theories, another dimension of their critical thinking.

Case study may be completed as an individual assignment and evaluated similarly to other written assignments, as long as the underlying reasoning process is assessed by the teacher. The earlier discussion of problem solving, decision making, and critical thinking, combined with questions for assessing critical thinking in Table 7.1, provide a framework for determining criteria for evaluation of the case study. The results of the case analysis may be presented orally for group critique and feedback. Lowenstein and Sowell (1992) also noted that case studies provide a strategy for integrating learning across courses and preparing students for the realities of their future practice.

DISCUSSION

Discussions with students individually and in small groups are an important strategy for evaluating problem-solving, decision-making, and critical-thinking abilities. In a discussion, the teacher has an opportunity to ask careful questions about students' thinking and the rationale they used for arriving at decisions and positions about issues. Discussions may be impromptu, for formative evaluation, or structured by the teacher who provides the context and questions to which students respond. Use of discussion for evaluating cognitive skills, however, requires careful questioning with a focus on the critical thinking used by students to arrive at answers. In these discussions, the teacher can ask students about possible decisions, reasons underlying each decision, consequences and implications of options they considered as part of their decision making, and different points of view in the situation. The level of questions asked, however, is significant to avoid a predominance of factual questions and focus on clarifying and higher level questions.

Questions. Factual questions are low-level, asking students to recall facts and specific information relative to the problem and issue being discussed, such as, "What is a stressor?""What are coping mechanisms?" Clarifying and explanatory questions require further thought and discussion. For instance, a clarifying question is, "Discuss the three stages of the general adaptation syndrome, responses in each stage, and observations you would make of the patient." For these questions, students explain their answers using their own terminology. Higher level questions, geared toward critical thinking, can not be answered by memory alone, require an evaluation or judgment of the situation, and may require comparisons (de Tornyay & Thompson, 1987). For instance, "What are similarities and differences between Selye's general adaptation syndrome and Lazarus' stress and coping theory?"Or, "Which pain intervention would you propose for this patient? Describe the underlying rationale for this intervention and alternate approaches possible."

Questions for discussions should be sequenced from low- to high-level, beginning with factual questions to evaluate students' knowledge of relevant concepts and theories and ability to apply them to the situation, problem, and issue, and progressing to questions that evaluate students' critical thinking. Wink (1993) proposed using Bloom's taxonomy as a framework for developing questions for discussions focusing on critical thinking. With this schema, low-level questions would ask for recall of facts and comprehension. Higher-level questions would focus on application, analysis, synthesis, and evaluation. This taxonomy of the cognitive domain was described and examples provided of each level in chapter 1.

This discussion of the level of questions asked by the teacher is important, for research suggests that teachers by nature do not ask higher-level questions of students.Questions asked of nursing students tend to focus on recall and comprehension, rather than higher levels of thinking (Craig & Page, 1981; Wang & Blumberg, 1983; Wink, 1995). Oermann (1996) concluded from a review of research in this area that discussions in nursing education tended to focus on recall and memorization of information and did not stimulate analytical thinking, ability to make judgments and consider multiple perspectives, and critical thinking in general. If discussions are to be geared toward evaluation of problem solving, decision making and critical thinking, the teacher needs an awareness of the level of questions asked for this purpose. Wink (1995) suggested that careful questioning enabled students to apply previously acquired knowledge to a situation, analyze problems and solutions, and develop critical-thinking and problem-solving skills, among other benefits.

The questions presented in Table 7.1 for evaluating critical thinking may be used to guide discussions. In a discussion, ask students about:

- *the purposes and goals* to be met;
- *questions, issues, and problems* to be resolved;
- *assumptions* on which their thinking is based;
- their own *points of view* and those of others;
- *information and evidence* on which they are basing their thinking;
- *concepts and theories* applicable to the question, issue, or problem being discussed;
- *inferences and conclusions* possible; and
- *implications and consequences* of their reasoning.

Socratic Method. The Socratic method also may be used for developing questions to evaluate students' critical thinking in a discussion. There are two phases in the Socratic method: systematic questioning and drawing comparisons. In systematic questioning, the initial phase, the teacher designs a series of questions that leads students along predetermined paths to rational thinking (Overholser, 1992).Questions are open-ended, have multiple possibilities for responding, offer different points of view, and ask students to defend their views and positions. In the Socratic method, the teacher avoids questions with one correct answer. In the second phase of questioning, the teacher directs students to draw comparisons and generalizations from the situation being analyzed to others.

Paul (1993) summarized the purpose of Socratic questions as raising issues for analysis, probing beneath the surface, and pursuing problematic areas of thinking. He suggested four types of Socratic discussions appropriate for evaluating critical thinking:

1. Exploratory discussions about complex issues in which students divide the issue into parts for analysis; explore individually one part of the issue; and then share, analyze, and evaluate their work in a follow-up discussion.
2. Fishbowl discussions in which one-third of the class, sitting in a circle, discusses an issue or controversial topic. The remainder of the class, positioned in a circle around the discussion group, then critiques the discussion from a critical thinking perspective.
3. Essay items in which students respond to a point of view expressed in a discussion.
4. Written summaries students complete immediately following a discussion adding new thoughts and perspectives. (p. 341)

DEBATE

Debate provides an effective mechanism for evaluating students' ability to analyze problems and issues in depth, consider alternate points of view, formulate a position to be taken after analyzing opposing viewpoints, and develop a rationale for decisions. In a debate, students develop an argument for or against a particular position or stand on an issue. "To persuade the audience to accept or reject a given position, debaters provide reasoned arguments for or against a matter of concern"(Garrett, Schoener, & Hood, 1996, p. 37). The process of formulating the issue for the debate, considering alternate viewpoints, and preparing arguments for a position taken provides an opportunity for assessment of students' critical-thinking skills.

In evaluating debates and oral presentations of an argument, Nitko (1996) recommended considering seven factors:

Did the student:

1. State clearly and enthusiastically the main point of the analysis?
2. Define clearly and effectively key terms and concepts?

3. Use sound reasoning to support the position taken?
4. Give appropriate facts that support the position?
   - Draw appropriate generalizations from the facts?
   - Have credible evidence?
   - Use the facts effectively in making the argument?
5. Evaluate alternate positions fairly?
   - Consider all relevant and important alternate positions?
   - Evaluate each one?
6. Rebut the alternate positions effectively?
   - Consider their inadequacies?
   - Convince the audience?
7. Present a well organized argument?
   - Keep audience interested and focused on main issues? (p. 206)

MULTIMEDIA

Multimedia may be used to present a scenario for problem solving, decision making, and critical thinking. Media add to the reality of the situation in comparison with presentation in a written format. Any type of media may be used for this purpose. Segments from videotapes present real-life scenarios to ask students about; questions may focus on identifying problems seen in the videotape, alternate problems to be considered, approaches that may be used and consequences of each, and varied decisions possible. Students also may be asked to identify their own beliefs, values, and feelings that may influence their interpretation of the videotape and decision making. Alternate perspectives may be considered, and students may be asked to take a stand and provide support for it. Audiotapes may be used to evaluate skills in analyzing interactions, identifying values and beliefs implied in responses, and proposing strategies for responding. Typically the media clip should be short, about 1 to 3 minutes, for students to remember what they see and hear (Reilly & Oermann, 1990).

Computer-assisted instruction (CAI), and particularly computer simulations, are another type of multimedia appropriate for evaluating higher level cognitive skills. With CAI, students may be presented with a problem to be solved and decisions to be made; some CAI is designed to provide students with feedback regarding the outcomes of their decisions. In interactive video, the computer simulation is combined with videotape or videodisk; students view the video of a scenario and respond to questions presented by the computer. While many of the commercially available CAI and interactive videos are effective for evaluating higher-level cognitive skills, particularly in a group format, questions typically need to accompany them to assess the underlying thought process for arriving at answers.

SHORT WRITTEN ASSIGNMENTS

Evaluation of written assignments is presented in chapter 6. For the purposes of assessing critical-thinking and other cognitive skills, however, these written assignments need to reflect additional principles. Assignments for this purpose should be short and should focus on an aspect of problem solving, decision making, and critical thinking. Long term papers often require summarization and synthesis of the literature, with only minimal critical and independent thinking. Meyers (1986) suggested that term papers are frequently exercises in summarizing the thoughts of others, rather than reflections of students' own thinking. As a result, students report on the ideas of others; they may not necessarily consider different problems and solutions possible, alternate points of view, issues to be addressed, and the other dimensions of critical thinking discussed earlier.

Short written assignments, in contrast, provide an opportunity for students to express their critical thinking in writing and for faculty to give prompt feedback to them on their reasoning. Meyers (1986) suggested that written assignments for evaluating critical thinking should meet the following criteria:

1. They should be short assignments focusing on some dimension of critical thinking.
2. A series of writing assignments for this purpose should build on one another, providing for the development of skill in thinking.
3. Beginning written assignments should ask students to recognize a problem or issue, identify key concepts, and ask questions to clarify it further.
4. Subsequent assignments should focus on recognizing assumptions, critiquing arguments, taking a stand and developing a rationale to support it, and other more complex critical thinking abilities.
5. Assignments should focus on real questions, problems, and issues, promoting transfer of learning to the practice setting.
6. The teacher should provide clear directions to guide student analysis and writing.

Examples of written assignments for assessing critical thinking, appropriate for either formative or summative evaluation, include short papers (one to two pages):

- Comparing different data sets;
- Comparing problems and alternate approaches possible;
- Analyzing issues, alternate courses of actions that could be used, and why each one would be effective;
- Analyzing different points of view, perspectives, and positions on an issue;
- Comparing a student's own and others' points of view on an issue or topic;
- Presenting evidence on which their reasoning is based;
- Analyzing conclusions drawn, evidence to support these conclusions, and alternate ones possible given the same evidence; and
- Presenting an argument to support a position.

Nitko's (1996) factors for evaluating debates and oral presentations of an argument also apply to evaluating the quality of written assignments in which an argument is presented to support a position.

INSTRUMENTS FOR MEASURING CRITICAL THINKING

There are a number of instruments available for measuring critical thinking among nursing students, although none of these instruments is specific to nursing education. A brief description is provided of each of these tests.

1. *Watson-Glaser Critical Thinking Appraisal (WGCTA)*. The WGCTA is the most widely used instrument for measuring critical thinking in nursing (Adams, Whitlow, Stover, & Johnson, 1996; Beck, Bennett, McLeod, & Molyneaux, 1992). It is designed to measure critical thinking as a general ability. Consisting of 80 items, the WGCTA has five subtests, with 16 items each, to measure ability to discriminate among truthful and untruthful inferences, recognize assumptions, deduce if conclusions follow the data, interpret information to determine if conclusions and generalizations are valid, and evaluate arguments (Watson & Glaser, 1980). The WGCTA tests logic and reasoning skill. Reliability was determined in several ways. Alpha coefficients ranged from 0.69 to 0.85; test-retest reliability was 0.73. In one review of research on critical thinking in nursing, 12 out of 13 nursing studies used the WGCTA as one of the dependent measures (Beck et al., 1992). Adams et al.(1996) summarized the findings from their review of nursing education research using the WGCTA. They reported a positive correlation between critical thinking and NCLEX–RN scores, but inconsistent findings in the areas of clinical judgment, levels of educational preparation, and changes in critical thinking from entry to and exit from the nursing program.

2. *California Critical Thinking Skills Test (CCTST)* . The California Critical Thinking Skills Test describes critical thinking as purposeful, self-regulatory judgment resulting in interpretation, analysis, evaluation, inference, explanation, and self-regulation (Facione, 1992; Facione & Facione, 1996). The CCTST addresses areas of analysis, evaluation, inference, and inductive and deductive reasoning. There are 34 items in multiple-choice format. Kuder-Richardson reliability was estimated as 0.68 to 0.69. Concurrent, content, and construct validity were established through a series of studies (Adams et al., 1996).

3. *California Critical Thinking Dispositions Inventory (CCTDI).* The California Critical Thinking Dispositions Inventory measures students' dispositions toward critical thinking. The dispositional dimension of critical thinking reflects a "critical spirit," attitudes that represent a "personal disposition to prize and to use critical thinking in one's personal, professional, and civic affairs" (Facione, Facione, & Sanchez, 1994, p. 345). One assumption underlying the development of the Dispositions Inventory is that critical thinking requires more than skills alone; the individual needs a disposition to value and use critical thinking. There are seven CCTDI disposition subscales:open-mindedness, analyticity, cognitive maturity, truth-seeking, systematicity, inquisitiveness, and self-confidence. Cronbach's alpha was 0.92; correlation with the California Critical Thinking Skills Test was 0.66 and 0.67 (Facione et al., 1994).

4. *Ennis-Weir Critical Thinking Essay Test (EWCTET).* The Ennis-Weir Test uses essay items to measure critical thinking. The intent is to measure the degree to which the student can "evaluate a given argument in the format of a written essay" (Adams et al., 1996, p. 29). There are different aspects of critical thinking evaluated: getting the point, identifying reasons and assumptions, stating one's point, offering reasons for it, seeing other possibilities, and responding to arguments (Ennis & Weir, 1985). Rane-Szostak and Robertson (1996) suggested that since scores are dependent on judgments made by examiners, interrater reliability is a concern.

5. *Cornell Critical Thinking Test (CCTT) Levels X and Z.* The CCTT measures a variety of critical thinking skills; these include induction, deduction, value judgment, observation, credibility, assumptions, and meaning. Internal consistency ranged from 0.67 to 0.90 for one form (Level X for 4th grade through second-year college students) and 0.50 to 0.77 for the second form (Level Z for gifted high-school students, college-aged students, and adults (Adams et al., 1996). Adams et al.(1996) suggested that the Cornell Critical Thinking and Ennis-Weir Critical Thinking Essay Tests have "untapped potential" and should be considered for testing in nursing.

While standardized instruments for measuring critical thinking in nursing are available, further research is indicated to test their use for different levels of nursing students. In addition, studies need to build on one another, rather than representing research with one group of students in one setting only. As research on the use of the California Critical Thinking Skills Test and California Critical Thinking Dispositions Inventory with nursing students becomes available, faculty will need to review these studies prior to deciding on instruments to use for measuring critical thinking in nursing.

SUMMARY

This chapter provided a framework for evaluating higher level cognitive skills, problem solving, decision making, and critical thinking among nursing students. In the practice setting, students are faced with client and other problems to be solved. Some of these problems relate to managing client, family, and community health needs; others involve problems associated with one's role and work environment. Ability to solve client- and setting-related problems is an essential skill to be developed and evaluated. Problem solving begins with recognizing and defining the problem, gathering data to clarify it further, developing solutions, and evaluating their effectiveness.

The nurse continually makes decisions about problems, solutions, alternate approaches that might be possible, and the best approach to use in a particular situation. Other decisions are needed for delivering care, managing the clinical environment, and carrying out other activities. In decision making, the learner arrives at a decision after considering a number of alternatives and weighing the consequences of each.

Critical thinking is reflective and reasoned thinking about nursing problems without one solution, focused on decisions about what to believe and do. There are eight elements of reasoning to be considered in the process of critical thinking that are applicable to evaluating critical thinking among nursing students. Strategies were presented for incorporating these elements of reasoning within the evaluation protocol for critical thinking.

In evaluating these cognitive skills, the teacher as a basic principle introduces new or novel material for analysis. Without the introduction of new material as part of the evaluation, students may have memorized from prior discussion or their readings how to problem solve and arrive at decisions for the situation at hand; they may recall the typical problem and solutions without thinking through alternate possibilities themselves. As a result, an essential component of this type of evaluation is the introduction of new information not encountered by the student at an earlier point in the instruction. In nursing, this is frequently accomplished by developing scenarios that present a novel situation for students to apply concepts and theories, problem solve, arrive at decisions, and in general engage in critical thinking. These items are referred to as context-dependent item sets or interpretative exercises. In a context-dependent item set, the teacher presents introductory material that students then analyze and answer questions about. The introductory material may be a description of a clinical situation, patient data, research findings, issues associated with clinical practice, and varied types of scenarios; students then read, analyze, and interpret this material and answer questions about it or complete other tasks.

Other methods for evaluating cognitive skills in nursing were presented in the chapter: case method and study, discussions using higher level and Socratic questioning, debate, multimedia, short written assignments designed specifically for evaluating critical thinking and other cognitive skills, and standardized tests for critical thinking. In addition to these strategies, clinical evaluation methods that provide for an assessment of cognitive skills are presented in chapter 11.

REFERENCES

Adams, M. H., Whitlow, J. F., Stover, L. M., & Johnson, K. W.(1996). Critical thinking as an educational outcome: An evaluation of current tools of measurement. *Nurse Educator, 21*(3), 23–32.

American Nurses Association. (1985). *Code for nurses with interpretive statements.* Kansas City, MO: Author.

American Nurses Association. (1995). *Nursing's social policy statement.* Washington, DC: Author.

Beck, S. E., Bennett, A., McLeod, R., & Molyneaux, D. (1992). Review of research on critical thinking in nursing education. In L. R. Allen (Ed.), *Review of research in nursing education* (Vol. V, pp. 1–30). New York: National League for Nursing.

Benner, P. (1984). *From novice to expert: Excellence and power in clinical nursing practice.* Menlo Park, CA: Addison-Wesley.

Case, B. (1994). Walking around the elephant: A critical-thinking strategy for decision making. *Journal of Continuing Education in Nursing, 25,* 101–109.

Craig, J. L., & Page, G.(1981). The questioning skills of nursing instructors. *Journal of Nursing Education, 20,* 18–23.

de Tornyay, R., & Thompson, M. A. (1987). *Strategies for teaching nursing* (3rd ed.). New York: John Wiley.

Ennis, R. H., & Weir, E. (1985). *The Ennis-Weir Critical Thinking Essay Test.* Pacific Grove, CA: Midwest Publications.

Facione, P.(1992). *The California Critical Thinking Skills Test: Forms A and B.* Millbrae, CA: California Academic Press.

Facione, N. C., & Facione, P. (1996). Externalizing the critical thinking in knowledge development and clinical judgment. *Nursing Outlook, 44*, 129–136.

Facione, N. C., Facione, P., & Sanchez, C. A. (1994). Critical thinking disposition as a measure of competent clinical judgment: The development of the California Critical Thinking Disposition Inventory. *Journal of Nursing Education, 33*, 345–350.

Foundation for Critical Thinking. (1994). *Critical thinking workshops.* Santa Rosa, CA: Author.

Fuszard, B. (1995). Case method. In B. Fuszard (Ed.), *Innovative teaching strategies in nursing* (2nd ed., pp. 81–92). Gaithersburg, MD: Aspen.

Garrett, M., Schoener, L., & Hood, L. (1996). Debate: A teaching strategy to improve verbal communication and critical-thinking skills. *Nurse Educator, 21*(4), 37–40.

Hursh, B., Haas, P. & Moore, M. (1983). An interdisciplinary model to implement general education. *Journal of Higher Education, 54*, 42–59.

Kataoka-Yahiro, M., & Saylor, C. (1994). A critical thinking model for nursing judgment. *Journal of Nursing Education, 33*, 351–356.

Kintgen-Andrews, J. (1991). Critical thinking and nursing education: Perplexities and insights. *Journal of Nursing Education, 30*, 152–157.

Lowenstein, A. J., & Sowell, R. (1992). Clinical case studies: A strategy for teaching leadership and management. *Nurse Educator, 17*(5), 15–18.

Meyers, C. (1986). *Teaching students to think critically.* San Francisco: Jossey-Bass.

Nitko, A. J. (1996). *Educational assessment of students* (2nd ed.). Englewood Cliffs, NJ: Prentice Hall.

Oermann, M. H. (1996). Research on teaching in the clinical setting. In K. P. Stevens (Ed.), *Review of research in nursing education* (Vol. VIII, pp. 91–126). New York: National League for Nursing.

Oermann, M. H. (1997). Evaluating critical thinking in clinical practice. *Nurse Educator, 22*(5), 25–28.

Overholser, J. C. (1992). Socrates in the classroom. *College Teaching, 40*(1), 14–19.

Paul, R. W. (1993). *Critical thinking: How to prepare students for a rapidly changing world.* Santa Rosa, CA: Foundation for Critical Thinking.

Perry, W. G., Jr. (1970). *Forms of intellectual and ethical development in the college years.* New York: Holt, Rinehart & Winston.

Rane-Szostak, D., & Robertson, J. F. (1996). Issues in measuring critical thinking: Meeting the challenge. *Journal of Nursing Education, 35*, 5–11.

Reilly, D. E., & Oermann, M. H. (1992). *Clinical teaching in nursing education* (2nd ed.). New York: National League for Nursing.

Reilly, D. E., & Oermann, M. H. (1990). *Behavioral objectives: Evaluation in nursing* (3rd ed.). New York: National League for Nursing.

Wang, A. M., & Blumberg, P. (1983). A study on interaction techniques of nursing faculty in the clinical area. *Journal of Nursing Education, 22*, 144–150.

Watson, G., & Glaser, E. M. (1980). *Watson-Glaser critical thinking appraisal manual.* Cleveland, OH: Psychological Corporation.

Wink, D. M. (1993). Using questioning as a teaching strategy. *Nurse Educator, 18*(5), 11–15.

Wink, D. M. (1995). The effective clinical conference. *Nursing Outlook, 43*, 29–32.

8

Assembling and Administering Tests

In addition to the preparation of a test blueprint and the skillful construction of test items to which it corresponds, the final appearance of
the test and the way in which it is administered can affect the validity of
the test results. A haphazard arrangement of test items, confusing or absent
directions, and typographical errors may contribute to measurement error
(Nitko, 1996). By following certain design rules, teachers can avoid such
errors when assembling a test.

Administering a test is usually the simplest phase of the testing process.
There are some common problems associated with test administration,
however, that also may affect the reliability and validity of the resulting
scores. Careful planning can help the teacher to avoid or minimize such
difficulties. This chapter discusses the process of assembling the test and
administering it to students.

TEST DESIGN RULES

Allow Enough Time

As discussed in chapter 3, preparing a high-quality test requires time for
the design phases as well as for the item-writing phase. Assembling the
test is not simply a clerical or technical task; the teacher should make all
decisions about the arrangement of test elements and the final appearance
of the test, even if someone else types or prints the test. The teacher must

allow enough time for this phase to avoid errors that could affect students' test scores (Gaberson, 1996).

Arrange Test Items in a Logical Sequence

Various methods for ordering items on the test have been recommended, including arrangement in order of difficulty and according to the sequence in which content was taught (Ebel & Frisbie, 1991, p. 205; Nitko, 1996, p. 301). However, if the test contains items of 2 or more formats, the teacher first should group items of the same format together. Since each item format requires different tasks of the student, this type of arrangement makes it easier for students to maintain the mental set required to answer each type of item, and prevents errors caused by frequent changing of task. Keeping items of the same format together also facilitates scoring if a scannable answer sheet is not used (Gaberson, 1996; Mehrens & Lehmann, 1991, p. 153).

Within each item-format group, items may be arranged to begin with the easiest items and progress in difficulty. Even well-prepared students are likely to be somewhat anxious at the beginning of a test, and encountering difficult items may increase their anxiety and interfere with their optimum performance. Beginning with easy items may build students' confidence and allow them to answer these items quickly and reserve more time for difficult items. Another method for arranging items is according to the order in which the content was taught, which may assist students to recall information more easily. The teacher can easily combine the difficulty and content-sequence methods of ordering items within each item-format section of the test (Gaberson, 1996; Nitko, 1996, p. 301).

Write Directions

The teacher cannot assume that students know the basis on which they are to select or provide answers, or how and where to record their answers to test items. As Mehrens and Lehmann (1973) pointed out, "You might have a car that is well tuned, aligned, has good tires and a battery, but it will be of little use to you in reaching your destination if you do not know in what direction to drive" (p. 313). Similarly, students may be well prepared, rested, and confident, but unable to perform at their best if the teacher does not tell them what to do (Gaberson, 1996).

The test should begin with a set of clear general directions that include instructions on how and where to record responses, what type of writing implement to use, whether or not students may write on the test booklet, the amount of time allowed, the number of pages and items on the exam, the types and point value of items, whether students may ask questions during the test, and what to do after finishing the exam (Ebel & Frisbie, 1991; Gaberson, 1996; Klisch, 1994; Nitko, 1996). Students may need to know some of these instructions while they are preparing for the test, for instance, if their answers to items requiring them to supply the names of medications must be spelled accurately in order to be scored as correct (Gaberson, 1996).

Each item-format section should begin with specific instructions. For multiple-choice items, the student needs to know whether to select the correct or best response. Directions for completion and essay items should state whether spelling, grammar, punctuation, and organization will be considered in scoring. For computation items, directions should specify the degree of precision required, the unit of measure, whether to show the calculation work, and what method of computation to use if there is more than one. Matching exercise directions should clearly specify the basis on which the match is to be made (Ebel & Frisbie, 1991; Gaberson, 1996).

Use a Cover Page

The general test directions may be printed on a cover page (Figure 8.1). A cover page also serves to keep the test items hidden from view during the distribution of the exam, so that the first students to receive the test will not have more time to complete it than students who receive their copies later (Ebel & Frisbie, 1991, p. 204; Nitko, 1996, p. 301). If the directions on the cover page indicate the number of pages and items, students can quickly check their test booklets for completeness and correct sequence of pages. The teacher then can replace defective test booklets before students begin answering items (Gaberson, 1996).

When a separate answer sheet is used, the cover page may be numbered to help maintain test security; students are directed to record this number on the answer sheet. After the test, the teacher can track any missing test booklets (Cangelosi, 1990).

Avoid Crowding

Test items are difficult to read when they are crowded together on the page; learning-disabled students and those for whom English is a second language may find crowding particularly trying. Techniques that allow students to read efficiently and to prevent errors in recording their responses include leaving sufficient white space within and between items

Exam Number_____

PSYCHIATRIC–MENTAL HEALTH
NURSING FINAL EXAM

Directions

1. This test consists of 12 pages. Please check your test booklet to make sure you have the correct number of pages in the proper sequence.
2. Parts I and II consist of 86 multiple-choice and matching items. You may write on the test booklet but **you must record your answers to these items on your answer sheet**. This part of the test will be machine-scored; read carefully and follow the instructions below:

    a. Use a #2 pencil.
    b. Notice that the items on the answer sheet are numbered **DOWN** the page in each column.
    c. Choose the **ONE BEST** response to each item. Items with multiple answer marks will be counted as incorrect. Fill in the circle completely; if you change your answer, erase your first answer thoroughly.
    d. Print your name (last name, first name) in the blocks provided, then fill in completely the corresponding circle in each column. If you wish to have your score posted, fill in an identification number of up to 9 digits (**DO NOT** use your Social Security Number) and fill in the corresponding circle in each column.
    e. Above your name, write your test booklet number.

3. Part III consists of 2 essay items. Directions for this section are found on page 12. Write your answers to these items on the lined paper provided. You may use pen or pencil. On each page of your answers, write your **TEST BOOKLET NUMBER. DO NOT** write your name on your answers.

4. If you have a question during the test, do not leave your seat — raise your hand and a proctor will come to you.

5. You have until 11:00 a.m. to complete this test.

Figure 8.1 Example of a cover page with general directions.

and indenting certain elements (Ebel & Frisbie, 1991; Klisch, 1994). Tightly packing words on a page may minimize the amount of paper used for testing, but facilitating maximum student performance on a test is worth a small additional expense for a few more sheets of paper (Gaberson, 1996).

Optimum spacing varies for each item format. The response options for a multiple-choice item should not be printed in tandem fashion, as the following example illustrates:

1. Which method of anesthesia involves injection of an agent into a nerve bundle which supplies the operative site?

A. General;   B. Local;   C. Regional;   D. Spinal;   E. Topical

The options are much easier to read if listed in a single column below the stem (Ebel & Frisbie, 1991, pp. 174, 204; Nitko, 1996, p. 147), as in this example:

Which method of anesthesia involves injection of an agent into a nerve bundle which supplies the operative site?
   a. General
   b. Local
   c. Regional
   d. Spinal
   e. Topical

Notice in this example that the second line of the stem is indented to the same position as the first line, and that the responses are slightly indented. This spacing makes the item number and its content easier to read (Gaberson, 1996).

Keep Related Material Together

The stem of a multiple-choice item and all related responses should appear on the same page. Both columns of a matching exercise also should be printed side by side and on one page, including the related directions; using short lists of premises and responses makes this arrangement easier. With context-dependent items, the introductory material and all related items should be contained on the same page, if possible. Otherwise, students may be distracted as they turn pages back and forth to read and respond to the test items, and they may make careless errors unrelated to their knowledge of the content (Nitko, 1996, pp. 156, 178).

Facilitate Scoring

If the test will be scored by hand, the layout of the test or the answer sheet should facilitate easy scoring. A separate answer sheet can be constructed to permit rapid scoring by comparing student responses to an answer key. If students record their answers directly on the test booklet, the test items should be arranged with scoring in mind. For example, a series of true-false items should be organized with columns of Ts and Fs at either the right or left margin so that students need only circle their responses, as in the following example:

T F   1. A stethoscope is required to perform auscultation.

T F   2. Physical exam techniques should be performed in the order of least to most intrusive.

T F   3. When using percussion, it is easier to detect a change from dullness to resonance.

Circling a letter, rather than writing or printing it, will prevent misinterpretation of students' handwriting. With completion items, printing blank spaces for the answers in tandem, as in the following example, makes scoring difficult:

1. List 3 responsibilities of the circulating nurse during induction of general anesthesia.

_____ ,   _____ ,   _____ ,

Instead, the blanks should be arranged in a column along one side of the page, as in this example:

1–3. List 3 responsibilities of the circulating nurse   1._____
during induction of general anesthesia.   2._____
3._____

Arrange the Correct Answers in a Random Pattern

There is a tendency for some teachers to favor certain response choices for the correct or keyed answer to objective test items, for example, to assign the correct response to the A or D position of a multiple-choice item. Some teachers arrange test items so that the correct answers form a pattern that makes scoring easy (e.g., T-F-T-F, or A-B-C-D). Test-wise students may use such test characteristics to gain an unfair advantage (Ebel & Frisbie, 1991; Gaberson, 1996). Response positions should be used with approximately equal frequency; there are several ways to accomplish this.

Many item-analysis software programs calculate the number of times the keyed response occurs in each position, or the teacher can tally the number of Ts and Fs, or As, Bs, Cs, and Ds, on the answer key by hand. For true-false items, if true or false statements are found to predominate, some items may be rewritten to make the distribution more equal (although it is recommended by some experts to include more false than true items). If the position of the correct response to multiple-choice items is determined by random assignment, each response position will be used approximately the same number of times (Ebel & Frisbie, 1991, pp. 149, 204).

Another way to arrange response alternatives for multiple-choice and matching items is according to a logical or meaningful order, such as alphabetical or chronological order, or in order of size or degree. This type of arrangement reduces reading and search time and helps knowledgeable students to locate the correct answer (Nitko, 1996, p. 148). This strategy also tends to randomly distribute the correct answer position, especially on lengthy tests (Gaberson, 1996).

Number the Items Continuously Throughout the Test

Although test items should be grouped according to format, they should be numbered continuously throughout the test. That is, the teacher should not start each new item format section with item number 1, but should continue numbering items in continuous sequence. This numbering system helps students to find items they may have skipped and to avoid making errors when recording their answers (Gaberson, 1996).

Proofread

The test items and directions should be free of spelling, punctuation, grammatical, and typing errors. Such defects are a source of measurement error and can cause confusion, distraction, and annoyance, particularly among learning-disabled students and those for whom English is a second language (Klisch, 1994). Often the test designer may not recognize his or her own errors; another teacher who knows the content may be asked to proofread a copy of the test before it is duplicated. The spell-check or grammar-check features of a word-processing program may not recognize punctuation errors or words that are spelled correctly but used in the wrong context, nor will they detect structural errors such as giving two test items the same number or two responses the same letter (Gaberson, 1996).

Prepare an Answer Key

Whether the test will be machine-scored or hand-scored, the teacher should prepare and verify an answer key in advance to facilitate efficient scoring and to provide a final check on the accuracy of the test items.

Scannable answer sheets also can be used for hand-scoring; an answer key can be produced by punching holes to indicate the correct answers. The teacher also should prepare ideal responses to essay items, identify intended responses to completion items, and make decisions regarding the point values of required answer elements if the analytical scoring method is used.

REPRODUCING THE TEST

Assure Legibility

Legibility is an important consideration when printing and duplicating the test; poor-quality copies may interfere with optimum student performance (Ebel & Frisbie, 1991, Nitko, 1996). A typeface that includes only upper-case letters is difficult to read; upper- and lower-case lettering is recommended. The master or original copy should be letter-quality, produced with a laser or bubble jet printer or a typewriter with a clean, carbon film ribbon; dot matrix print is unacceptable. For best results, the test should be photocopied on a machine that has sufficient toner to produce crisp, dark print. The glass surface of the photocopy machine should be cleaned to remove artifacts that will be copied onto the document (Gaberson, 1996).

Print on One Side of the Page

The test should be reproduced on only one side of each sheet of paper. Printing on both sides of each page could cause students to skip items unintentionally or make errors when recording their scores on a separate answer sheet. It also creates distractions from excessive page-turning during the test (Gaberson, 1996). If answers are recorded on the test booklet itself, printing on only one side will make hand-scoring easier (Mehrens & Lehmann, 1973).

Duplicate Enough Copies

For most tests, the teacher should duplicate enough copies so that each student has a copy (Ebel & Frisbie, 1991). Displaying test items on an overhead projector or writing them on the chalkboard may save money, but these procedures may cause problems for students with learning or visual disabilities. Under these conditions, students cannot control the pace at which they answer items or return to a previous item, and all test items cannot be displayed simultaneously unless it is a short quiz (Gaberson, 1996). In addition, once the chalkboard has been erased, there is no verifiable record of the wording of test items, which could present a problem if a student questions the scoring of an answer (Ebel & Frisbie, 1991, p. 203). Dictating test items is not recommended except when the objective is to test knowledge of correct spelling; in addition to creating problems for students with hearing impairments, this method wastes time that students could otherwise spend in thinking about and responding to the items. The teacher should duplicate more test copies than the number of students to allow for extra copies for proctors or replacement of defective copies that may have been distributed to students (Gaberson, 1996).

Maintain Test Security

Teachers have a serious responsibility to maintain the security of tests by protecting them from unauthorized access. Carelessness on the part of the teacher can permit dishonest students to gain access to test materials and use them to obtain higher grades than they deserve. This contributes to measurement error, and it is unfair to honest students who are well prepared for the test. Teachers should make arrangements to secure the test while it is being prepared, stored, administered, and scored (Gaberson, 1996).

Test materials should be stored in locked areas accessible only to authorized personnel. Computer files that contain test items should be protected with passwords, encryption, or similar security devices. Only regular employees should handle test materials; student employees should not be asked to type, print, or duplicate tests. While test items are being written or typed, they should be protected from the view of others by turning the monitor off or covering the typewriter if an unauthorized individual enters the area. Tests should be typed at times when the typist does not have to answer the telephone or attend to visitors (Gaberson, 1996).

One suggestion for preventing cheating during test administration to large groups is to prepare alternative forms of the test by arranging the same items in a different order (Ebel & Frisbie, 1991, Jenkins & Langley, 1991). Similarly, the order of responses to multiple-choice and matching items might be scrambled to produce an alternative form of the test. However, the psychometric properties of alternative forms produced in these ways might be sufficiently different as to result in different scores, especially when the positions of items with unequal difficulty are switched. If there is little or no evidence for the true equivalence of these alternative forms, teachers are advised not to use this approach (Gaberson,

1996); other ways to prevent cheating are discussed in the next section of this chapter.

TEST ADMINISTRATION

Environmental Conditions

The environmental conditions of test administration can be a source of measurement error if they interfere with students' performance. If possible, the teacher should select a room which limits potential distractions during the test. For example, if windows must be open for ventilation during warm weather, students may be distracted by lawn-mowing or construction noise; requesting a room on another side of the building may prevent the problem. The teacher also should try to avoid interruptions such as a fire alarm test or a disaster evacuation drill by asking the building manager to not schedule such events during the test. A sign such as "Testing—Quiet Please" on the door of the testing room may further reduce noise in the immediate area (Gaberson, 1996).

Distributing the Test Materials

Careful organization allows the teacher to distribute test materials and give instructions to the students efficiently. With large groups of students, several proctors may be needed to assist with this process. If a separate answer sheet is used, it usually can be distributed first, followed by the test booklets. During distribution of the test booklets, the teacher should instruct students to not turn the cover page and begin the test until told to do so. At this point, students should check their test booklets for completeness, and defective booklets are replaced. The teacher then should read the general directions aloud while students read along. Hearing the directions may help students whose anxiety may interfere with their comprehension of the written instructions. After answering any questions about test procedures, the teacher then tells students to turn the cover page and begin the test (Gaberson, 1996).

Answering Questions During the Test

Some students may find it necessary to ask questions of the teacher during a test, but responding to these questions is always somewhat disturbing to other students. Distraction can be kept to a minimum by telling students to raise their hands if they have questions, rather than leaving their seats to come to approach the teacher; a proctor then goes to each student's seat. Proctors should answer questions as quietly and briefly as possible. In answering questions, proctors certainly should address errors in the test copy and ambiguity in directions but should avoid giving clues to the correct answers. Students for whom English is not the native language may need additional help to understand general vocabulary or cultural information in test items (Ebel & Frisbie, 1991, pp. 205–206), although teachers should work to eliminate such cultural bias during the item-writing phase, as discussed in chapter 14.

Preventing Cheating

Cheating is widely believed to be common on college campuses in the United States, and even if the reported incidence is exaggerated, it "should not be allowed to establish cheating as an acceptable norm for student behavior or to persuade instructors that cheating is inevitable and must be accommodated as gracefully as possible" (Ebel & Frisbie, 1991, pp. 207–208).

Cheating is defined as any activity whose purpose is to gain a higher score on a test or other academic assignment than a student is likely to earn on the basis of achievement. Cheating on a test can take the form of acquiring test materials in advance of the test or sharing these materials with others, arranging for a substitute to take a test, preparing and using unauthorized notes during the test, exchanging information with others or copying answers from another student during the test, and copying test items or stealing test booklets to share with others who may take the test later. Teachers are responsible for avoiding conditions that make cheating easy, before, during, and after a test (Nitko, 1991). Students who do act honestly resent those who cheat, especially if dishonest students are rewarded with high test scores. Honest students also resent faculty who do not recognize and deal effectively with cheating (Gaberson, 1997).

Although a number of methods for preventing cheating during a test have been proposed, the single, most effective method is careful proctoring (Mehrens & Lehmann, 1991, p. 157). There should be enough proctors to supervise students adequately during exams; for most groups of students, at least two proctors are suggested so that one is available to leave the room with a student in case of emergency without leaving the remaining students unsupervised (Gaberson, 1996). Teachers should take seriously the task of proctoring tests and should devote their full attention to supervising students during the test instead of bringing other materials to work on during the exam (Ebel & Frisbie, 1991).

A particularly troubling situation for teachers is how to deal with a student's behavior during a test that suggests cheating. "If the teacher is satisfied beyond any reasonable doubt that a student is cheating, he or she needs no other justification for . . . collecting the examination materials and quietly dismissing the student from the room" (Ebel & Frisbie, 1991, p. 208). However, if it is possible that the teacher's interpretation of the behavior is incorrect, it may be best not to confront the student at that time. In addition to preventing a potentially innocent student from completing the test, confiscating test materials and ordering a student to leave will create a distraction to other students that may affect the validity of all students' test scores. A better response is to continue to observe the student, making eye contact if possible to make the student aware of the teacher's attention. If the student was attempting to cheat, this approach usually effectively stops the behavior. If the behavior continues, the teacher should attempt to verify this observation with another proctor, and if both agree, the student may be asked to leave the room (Gaberson, 1997). The appropriate penalty for cheating on a test is a score of zero for that test; merely deducting points from the student's score is not appropriate because the score should be considered invalid and no score recorded as if the student never took the test (Cangelosi, 1990).

If the teacher hears that a copy of a test is circulating in advance of the scheduled date of administration, the teacher should attempt to obtain verifiable evidence that some students have seen it. In this case, the only recourse is to prepare another test or use a different means to evaluate student achievement (Ebel & Frisbie, 1991).

Collecting Test Materials

When students are finished with the test and are preparing to leave the room, the resulting confusion and noise can disturb students who are still working. The teacher should plan for efficient collection of test materials to minimize such distractions and also to maintain test security. It is important to assure that no test materials leave the room with students. Therefore, teachers should take care to verify that students turn in their test booklets, answer sheets, scratch paper, and any other test materials. With a large group of students, one proctor may be assigned the task of collecting test materials from each student; this proctor should check the test booklet and answer sheet to assure that the directions for marking answers have been followed, that the student's name is recorded as directed, and that the student has not omitted any items. Any such errors can then be corrected before the student leaves the room, and test security will not be compromised.

If students are still working near the end of the allotted testing time, the remaining time should be announced and they should be encouraged to finish as quickly as possible. When time is called, students must stop their work and the teacher then collects all remaining tests (Ebel & Frisbie, 1991). In some cases, it may be appropriate to extend the testing time for students with legitimate learning disabilities, but this decision should be made in advance of the test and appropriate arrangements made.

SUMMARY

The final appearance of a test and the way in which it is administered can affect the validity of the test results. Poor arrangement of test items, confusing or absent directions, typographical errors, and careless administration may contribute to measurement error. Careful planning can help the teacher to avoid or minimize these difficulties.

Rules for good test design include allowing sufficient time, arranging test items in a logical sequence, writing general and item format directions, using a cover page, spacing test elements to avoid crowding, keeping related material together, arranging the correct answers in a random pattern, numbering items consecutively throughout the test, proofreading the test, and preparing an accurate answer key. In preparing to duplicate the test, the teacher should assure legibility, print the test on one side of each page, prepare enough copies for all students and proctors, and maintain the security of test materials.

Although administering a test is usually the simplest phase of the testing process, there are some common problems that may affect the reliability and validity of the resulting scores. Teachers should arrange for favorable environmental conditions, distribute the test materials and give directions efficiently, make appropriate plans for proctoring and answering questions during the test, and collect test materials efficiently. Teachers have an important responsibility to prevent cheating before, during, and after a test, and should respond to verified evidence of cheating with appropriate sanctions.

REFERENCES

Cangelosi, J. S. (1990). *Designing tests for evaluating student achievement*. New York: Longman.

Ebel, R. L., & Frisbie, D. A. (1991). *Essentials of educational measurement* (5th ed.). Englewood Cliffs, NJ: Prentice Hall.

Gaberson, K. B. (1997). Academic dishonesty. *Nursing Forum, 32* (3), 14–20.

Gaberson, K. B. (1996). Test design: Putting all the pieces together. *Nurse Educator, 21* (4), 28–33.

Jenkins, H. M., & Langley, C. G. (1991). A test protocol for large groups. *Nurse Educator, 16* (1), 8–10.

Klisch, M. L.(1994). Guidelines for reducing bias in nursing examinations. *Nurse Educator, 19* (2), 35–39.

Mehrens, W. A., & Lehmann, I. J. (1973). *Measurement and evaluation in education and psychology*. New York: Holt, Rinehart and Winston.

Mehrens, W. A. , & Lehmann, I. J. (1991). *Measurement and evaluation in education and psychology* (4th ed.). Fort Worth, TX: Holt, Rinehant and Winston.

Nitko, A. J. (1996). *Educational assessment of students* (2nd ed.). Englewood Cliffs, NJ: Prentice Hall.

9

Scoring and Analyzing Tests

A fter administering a test, the teacher's responsibility is to score it or arrange to have it scored. The teacher then interprets the results and uses these interpretations to make grading, selection, placement, or other decisions. In order to accurately interpret test scores, however, the teacher needs to analyze the performance of the test as a whole and of the individual test items, and to use these data to draw valid inferences about student performance. Information about how the test performed as a measurement tool also helps teachers to prepare for posttest discussions with students (Ebel & Frisbie, 1991). This chapter discusses the processes of obtaining scores and performing test and item analysis. It also suggests ways in which teachers can use posttest discussions to contribute to student learning and seek student feedback that can lead to test-item improvement.

SCORING

Many teachers say that they "grade" tests, when in fact it would be more accurate to say that they "score" tests. Scoring is the process of determining the first direct, unconverted, uninterpreted measure of performance on a test, usually called the raw score or observed score. The raw score represents the number of right answers (Mehrens & Lehmann, 1991). On the other hand, grading or marking is the process of assigning a symbol to represent the quality of the student's performance. Symbols can be letters (A, B, C, D, F; may also include + and -); categories (pass–fail, satisfactory–unsatisfactory); integers (9 through 1); or percentages (100, 99, 98 . . .), among other options (Nitko, 1996). In most cases, test scores should not be converted to grades for the purpose of later computing a final average grade. Instead, the teacher should record actual test scores and then combine them into a composite score that can be converted to a final grade. Recording scores contributes to greater measurement accuracy because information is lost each time scores are converted to grades. For example, if scores from 70 to 79 are all converted to a grade of C, each score in this range receives the same grade, although scores of 71 and 78 may represent important differences in achievement. If the C grades are all converted to the same numerical grade, for example, C = 2.0, then such distinctions are lost when the final composite score is calculated (Ebel & Frisbie, 1991, p. 279). Various grading systems and their uses are discussed in chapter 13.

Weighting Items

As a general rule, each objective-type test item should have equal weight. It is difficult for teachers to justify that one item is worth 2 points while another is worth 1 point; such a weighting system also motivates students to argue for partial credit for some answers. Differential weighting implies that the teacher believes knowledge of one concept to be more important than knowledge of another concept. If this is so, the teacher should sample the more important domain more heavily by writing more items in that area (Mehrens & Lehmann, 1991, p. 159).

Most machine-scoring systems assign 1 point to each correct answer; this seems reasonable for hand-scored tests as well. It is not necessary to adjust the numerical weight of items in order to achieve a total of 100 points. Although a test of 100 points allows the teacher to calculate a percentage score quickly, this step is not necessary to make valid interpretations of students' scores.

Correction for Guessing

The raw score sometimes is adjusted or corrected before it is interpreted. One procedure involves applying a formula intended to eliminate any advantage that a student might have gained by guessing correctly. The correction formula reduces the raw score by some fraction of the number of the student's wrong answers (Nitko, 1996, p. 307). The formula only can be used with true-false, multiple-choice, and some matching items, and is dependent upon the number of options per item. The general formula is :

$$\text{Corrected score} = R - \frac{W}{(n-1)} \qquad \text{[Equation 9.1]}$$

where R is the number of right answers, W is the number of wrong answers, and n is the number of options in each item (Nitko, 1996, p. 307). Thus, for 2-option items like true–false, the teacher merely subtracts the number of wrong answers from the number of right answers (or raw score); for 4-option items, the raw score is reduced by $^1/_3$ of the number of wrong answers. A correction formula obviously is difficult to use for a test that contains several different item formats.

The use of a correction formula is appropriate only when students have been instructed to not answer any item for which they are uncertain of the answer. Even under these circumstances, students may differ in their interpretation of "certainty" and therefore may interpret the advice differently. Some students will guess regardless of the instructions given and the threat of a penalty; the risk-taking or testwise student is likely to be rewarded with a higher score than the risk-avoiding or non-testwise student because of guessing some answers correctly. These personality differences cannot be equalized by instructions not to guess and penalties for guessing. The use of a correction formula also is based on the assumption that the student who does not know the answer will guess blindly. In fact, many students choose correct answers through intelligent informed guesses based on partial knowledge, and in these cases the formula undercorrects for guessing (Mehrens & Lehmann, 1991). Use of a correction formula also complicates the scoring process, allowing opportunities for clerical scoring errors (Nitko, 1996). Based on these limitations, the best approach is to advise all students to answer every item, and no correction for guessing should be applied.

ITEM ANALYSIS

Computer software for item analysis is widely available for use with electronic answer sheet scanning equipment. Figure 9.1 is an example of a computer-generated item analysis report. For teachers who do not have access to such equipment and software, procedures for analyzing student responses to test items by hand are described in detail later in this section. Regardless of the method used for analysis, teachers should be familiar enough with the meaning of each item analysis statistic to correctly interpret the results. It is important to realize that most item analysis techniques are designed for items that are scored dichotomously, that is, either right

ITEM STATISTICS (N = 68)									
Item	Key	A	B	C	D	E	Omit	Multiple response	Difficulty index	Discrimination index
1	A	44	0	24	0	0	0	0	.65	.34
2	B	0	62	4	2	0	0	0	.91	.06
3	A	59	1	4	4	0	0	0	.87	.35
4	C	12	4	51	1	0	0	0	.75	.19
5	E	23	8	0	8	29	0	0	.43	.21
6	D	2	3	17	46	0	0	0	.68	.17

Figure 9.1 Sample computer-generated item analysis report.

or wrong, from tests that are intended for norm-referenced uses (Ebel & Frisbie, 1991; Nitko, 1996).

Difficulty Index

One useful indication of test-item quality is its difficulty. The most commonly employed index of difficulty is the p level; p levels range from 0 to 1.00, indicating the percentage of students who answered the item correctly. A p value of 0 indicates that no one answered the item correctly, and a value of 1.00 indicates that every student answered the item correctly (Popham, 1990; Waltz, Strickland, & Lenz, 1991).

A simple formula for calculating the p value is:

$$p = \frac{R}{T} \qquad \text{[Equation 9.2]}$$

where R is the number of students who responded correctly and T is the total number of students who took the test (Nitko, 1996, p. 310; Popham, 1990, p. 273).

The difficulty index is commonly interpreted to mean that items with p values of .20 and below are difficult, and items with p values of .80 and above are easy. This interpretation may imply that test items are intrinsically easy or difficult, however, and may not take into account the quality of the instruction or the abilities of the students in that group. A group of students who were taught by an expert instructor might tend to answer a test item correctly, while a group of students with similar abilities who were taught by an ineffectual instructor might tend to answer it incorrectly. Different p values might be produced by students with more or less ability. It is clear from these examples that test items cannot be categorized automatically as "easy" or "difficult" without reference to the quality of teaching (Ebel & Frisbie, 1991; Popham, 1990).

The p value also should be interpreted in relationship to the student's probability of guessing the correct response. For example, if all students guess the answer to a true–false item, on the basis of chance alone the p value of that item should be approximately .50. On a 4-option multiple-choice item, chance alone should produce a p value of .25 (Popham, 1990, p. 274).

For most tests whose results will be interpreted in a norm-referenced way, p values of .30 to .70 are desirable. Very easy and very difficult items have little power to discriminate between students who know the content and students who do not, and they also decrease the reliability of the test scores (Ebel & Frisbie, 1991, p. 231; Waltz et al., 1991, p. 186). Teachers can use item-difficulty information to identify content that may need to be retaught or to identify test items that are ambiguous (Nitko, 1996).

Discrimination Index

The discrimination index, D, is a powerful indicator of test-item quality. A positively discriminating item is one that was answered correctly more often by students who scored well on the total test than by those who scored poorly on the total test. A negatively discriminating item was answered correctly more often by students who scored poorly on the test than by those who scored well. A nondiscriminating item is one for which there is no difference in the proportion of correct responders between high scoring and low scoring students (Popham, 1990).

A number of item discrimination indices are available; a simple method of computing D is:

$$D = p_h - p_l \qquad \text{[Equation 9.3]}$$

where p_h is the fraction of students in the high-scoring group who answered the item correctly and p_l is the fraction of students in the low-scoring group who answered the item correctly (Nitko, 1996, p. 313). Computer item analysis programs usually calculate D as a point biserial correlation coefficient between the total test score, a continuous variable, and performance on a specific item, scored dichotomously as correct or incorrect (Popham, 1990, p. 275).

The *D* value ranges from - 1.00 to + 1.00. In general, the higher the positive value, the better the test item. Ebel and Frisbie (1991) suggested that *D* values of .40 and higher indicate very good items, values between 0.30 and 0.39 indicate reasonably good items, values between .20 and .29 suggest that the item needs to be improved, and values below 0.19 indicate poor items that should be revised or not used again (p. 232). One possible interpretation of a negative *D* value is that the item was misinterpreted by high scorers (Waltz et al., 1991), who may have perceived a meaning in the item that the teacher did not intend to convey.

When interpreting a *D* value, it is important to keep in mind that an item's ability to discriminate is highly related to its difficulty index. An item that is answered correctly by all students has a difficulty index of 1.00; the discrimination index for this item is 0.00, because there is no difference in performance on that item between high scorers and low scorers. Similarly, if all students answered the item incorrectly, the difficulty index is 0.00, and the discrimination index is also 0.00 because there is no discrimination power (Popham, 1990). Negative *D* values signal items that should be reviewed carefully; they may need to be revised or eliminated (Nitko, 1996).

Distractor Analysis

As previously indicated, item-analysis statistics can serve as indicators of test-item quality. No teacher, however, should make decisions about retaining a test item in its present form, revising it, or eliminating it from future use on the basis of the item statistics alone. The teacher should carefully examine each questionable test item for evidence of poorly functioning distractors, ambiguous alternatives, and miskeying.

Every distractor should be selected by at least one lower-group student, and more lower-group students should select it than higher-group students. A distractor that is not selected by any student in the lower group may contain a technical flaw or may be so implausible as to be obvious even to students who lack knowledge of the correct answer. A distractor is ambiguous if upper-group students tend to choose it with about the same frequency as the keyed, or correct, response. This result usually indicates that there is no one clearly correct or best answer. Poorly functioning and ambiguous distractors may be revised to make them more plausible or to eliminate the ambiguity. If a large number of higher-scoring students select a particular wrong response, the teacher should check to see if the answer key is correct. In each case, the content of the item, not the statistics alone, should guide the teacher's decision making (Nitko, 1996, pp. 314–315).

Performing an Item Analysis by Hand

The following process for performing item analysis by hand is adapted from Ebel and Frisbie (1991), Nitko (1996), and Popham (1990):

Step 1. After the test is scored, arrange the test scores in rank order, highest to lowest.

Step 2. Divide the scores into a high-scoring half and a low-scoring half. For this step, some sources recommend dividing scores into equal thirds (Nitko, 1996, p. 309) or identifying scores in the upper and lower 25% of the distribution and not using the remaining scores for analysis (Ebel & Frisbie, 1991, p. 225; Waltz et al., 1991). The use of two groups is recommended for the purpose of this discussion because it is more useful with scores from small groups of students and because the resulting calculations are easy to perform.

Step 3. For each item, tally the number of students in each group who chose each alternative. Record these counts on a copy of the test item next to each response option. The keyed response for the following sample item is "d"; the group of 20 students is divided into 2 groups of 10 students each.

1. What is the most likely explanation for breast asymmetry in an adolescent girl ?

		Higher	Lower
a.	Blocked mammary duct in the larger breast	0	3
b.	Endocrine disorder	2	3
c.	Mastitis in the larger breast	0	0
*d.	Normal variation in growth	8	4

Step 4. Calculate the difficulty index for each item. The following formula is a variation of the one presented earlier, to account for the division of scores into two groups:

$$p = \frac{R_h + R_l}{T} \qquad \text{[Equation 9.4]}$$

where R_h is the number of students in the high-scoring half who answered correctly, R_l is the number of students in the low-scoring half who answered correctly, and T is the total number of students. For the purpose of calculating the difficulty index, consider omitted responses and multiple-responses as incorrect. For the example in Step 4, the p value is .60, indicating a moderately difficult item.

Step 5. Calculate the discrimination index for each item. Using the data from Step 4, divide R_h by the total number of students in that group to obtain p_h. Repeat the process to calculate p_l from R_l. Subtract p_l from p_h to obtain D, as in Equation 9.3. For the example in Step 4, the discrimination index is .40, indicating that the item discriminates well between high-scoring and low-scoring students.

Step 6. Check each item for implausible distractors, ambiguity, and miskeying. It is obvious that in the sample item, no students chose "Mastitis in the larger breast" as the correct answer. This distractor does not contribute to the discrimination power of the item, and the teacher should consider replacing it with an alternative that might be more plausible.

TEST CHARACTERISTICS

In addition to item analysis results, information about how the test performed as a whole also helps teachers to interpret test results. Measures of central tendency and variability, reliability estimates, and the shape of the score distribution can assist the teacher to make judgments about the quality of the test; difficulty and discrimination indices are related to these test characteristics. Test statistics are discussed in detail in chapter 12.

In addition, teachers should examine test items in the aggregate for evidence of bias. For example, although there may be no obvious gender bias in an any single test item, such a bias may be apparent when all items are reviewed as a group. Similar cases of racial, religious, and cultural bias may be detected and remedied when all items are examined together (Popham, 1990). The effect of bias on testing and evaluation is discussed in detail in chapter 14.

CONDUCTING POSTTEST DISCUSSIONS

Giving students feedback about test results can be an opportunity to reinforce learning, to correct misinformation, and to solicit their input for improvement of test items. A feedback session also can be an invitation to engage in battle, with students attacking to gain extra points and the teacher defending the honor of the test and, it often seems, the very right to give tests. Ebel and Frisbie (1991) suggested that posttest discussions can be beneficial to teachers and students alike if they are planned and conducted in a businesslike manner. The teacher should prepare for a posttest discussion by completing a test and item analysis and reviewing the items that were most difficult for the majority of students. The discussion should focus on the reasons why students answered these items incorrectly (Ebel & Frisbie, 1991). Student comments about test items, directions, and other test features can provide useful insights for teachers who are interested in improving their test construction abilities (Popham, 1990).

In order to use time efficiently, the teacher should give the correct answers quickly. If the test is hand-scored, correct answers may be indicated on the students' answer sheets or test booklets. If machine-scoring is used, the answer key may be reproduced on a transparency and displayed. Teachers should continue to protect the security of the test during the posttest discussion by accounting for all test booklets and answer sheets and by eliminating other opportunities for cheating. Some teachers do not allow students to use pens or pencils during the feedback session to prevent answer-changing and subsequent complaints that scoring errors were made. Another approach is to distribute pens with red or green ink and permit only those pens to be used to mark answers. Teachers also should decide in advance whether to permit students to take notes during the session.

One method for giving immediate posttest feedback to large groups of students was proposed by Jenkins and Langley (1991). Students record answers on both the answer sheet and the test booklet, both of which are identified with the students' names. As they finish the test, students submit their answer sheets to the proctor and leave their test booklets on their desks, face down. The answer sheets are then set aside for later scoring. When the testing period is over, students return to the room to review their answers. The teacher projects the correct answers onto a screen, and students compare them with the answers they marked in their test booklets. Although test items are not discussed at this time, students are given the opportunity to write questions or concerns about specific test items on feedback request sheets. The test booklets and feedback request sheets are then collected. Review of 50 to 75 test items can be accomplished in about 20 minutes. Feedback sheets are later returned to students with teacher comments; students who need additional help are encouraged to make appointments with the teacher for individual review sessions. Student feedback may also be used to make necessary item revisions (Jenkins & Langley, 1991). One disadvantage to this method of giving posttest feedback is that because the test has not yet been scored and analyzed, the teacher will not have an opportunity to thoroughly prepare for the session; feedback consists only of the correct answers, and no discussion takes place.

Whatever the structure of the posttest discussion, the teacher should control the session so that it produces maximum benefit for all students.

While discussing an item that was answered incorrectly by a majority of students, the teacher should maintain a calm, matter-of-fact, nondefensive attitude. Students who answered the item incorrectly may be asked to provide their rationale for choosing an incorrect response; students who supplied or chose the right answer may be asked to explain why it is correct. The teacher should avoid engaging in arguments with individual students that do not contribute substantively to the class discussion (Ebel & Frisbie, 1991); instead, the teacher should either invite written comments as described above or schedule individual appointments to discuss the items in question.

Eliminating Items or Adding Points

Teachers often debate the merits of adjusting test scores by eliminating items or adding points to compensate for real or perceived deficiencies in test construction or performance. For example, during a posttest discussion, students may argue that if they all answered an item incorrectly, the item should be omitted or all students should be awarded an extra point to compensate for the "bad item." It is interesting to note that students seldom propose subtracting a point from their scores if they all answer an item correctly. In any case, how should the teacher respond to such requests? In this discussion, a distinction is made between test items that are technically flawed and those that do not function as intended.

If test items are properly constructed, critiqued, and proofread, it is unlikely that serious flaws will appear on the test. However, errors that do appear may have varying effects on students' scores. For example, if the correct answer to a multiple-choice item is inadvertently omitted from the test, no student will be able to answer the item correctly. In this case, the item simply should not be scored. That is, if the error is discovered during or after the test is given and before it is scored, the item is omitted from the answer key; a test that was intended to be worth 73 points is then worth 72 points. If the error is discovered after the tests are scored, they can be rescored. Students often worry about the effect of this change on their scores and may argue that they should be awarded an extra point in this case. The possible effects of both adjustments on a hypothetical score are as follows:

	Total possible points	Raw score	Percentage correct
Original test	73	62	84.9
Flawed item not scored	72	62	86.1
Point added to raw score	73	63	86.3

It is obvious that omitting the flawed item and adding a point to the raw score produce nearly identical results. Although students might view adding a point to their scores as more satisfying, it makes little sense to award a point for an item that was not answered correctly. The "extra" point in fact does not represent knowledge of any content area or achievement of an objective, and therefore it does not contribute to a valid interpretation of the test scores. Teachers should inform students matter-of-factly that an item was eliminated from the test and reassure them that their relative standing with regard to performance on the test has not changed.

If the technical flaw consists of a misspelled word in a true-false item that does not change the meaning of the statement, no adjustment should be made. The teacher should avoid a lengthy debate about item semantics if it is clear that such errors are unlikely to have affected students' scores. Teachers should welcome such feedback from students, however, and use it to improve test items for future use (Ebel & Frisbie, 1991).

Teachers should resist the temptation to eliminate items from the test solely on the basis of low difficulty and discrimination indices. Omission of items may affect the validity of the scores from the test, particularly if several items related to one content area or objective are eliminated, resulting in inadequate sampling of that content (Flynn & Reese, 1988).

Because identified flaws in test construction do contribute to measurement error, the teacher should consider taking them into account when using the test scores to make grading decisions and set cut-off scores. That is, the teacher should not fix cut-off scores for assigning grades until after all tests have been given and analyzed. The proposed grading scale then can be adjusted if necessary to compensate for deficiencies in test construction. Students should be informed of the possibility that the grading scale may be adjusted in this way and reassured that the change would not affect their grades adversely (Ebel & Frisbie, 1991, p. 239).

DEVELOPING A TEST ITEM BANK

Since a great amount of effort usually goes into developing, administering, and analyzing test items, teachers should develop a system for maintaining and expanding a pool or bank of items from which to select items for future tests. Traditionally, item banks are maintained in file boxes or drawers, but microcomputers now allow teachers to maintain databases of test items on disks (Cangelosi, 1990).

For a file box system, each test item is printed on a separate index card; if the cards are 4" x 6" or larger, often the teacher can simply cut a test

Front of Card

Physical Assessment   Unit 5
                                                     Objective 3

1. What is the most likely explanation for breast asymmetry in
   an adolescent girl?

   a. Blocked mammary duct in the larger breast
   b. Endocrine disorder
   c. Mastitis in the larger breast
   *d. Normal variation in growth

Back of Card

Test date	Difficulty index	Discrimination index
10/22/95	.72	.25
2/20/96	.56	.33
10/24/96	.60	.40

Figure 9.2 Sample item card for a file box test bank.

booklet apart and mount each item on a separate card. The keyed, or correct, response is indicated for objective-type items. For completion or essay
items, a brief scoring key should be included. The test item can be coded
for the course, unit, content area, or objective for which it was designed.
The back of the card can be used to record a history of the item analysis
results. Figure 9.2 is an example of a card for the sample item discussed
above.

Commercially produced software programs can be used in a similar
way to develop a data base of test items. Each test item is a record in the
database. The test items then can be sorted according to the fields in which
the data are entered; for example, the teacher could retrieve all items that
are classified as Objective 3, with a moderate difficulty index.

Many publishers also offer test item banks that relate to the content
contained in their textbooks. Although some teachers would consider these
item banks to be a shortcut to the development and selection of test items,
they should be evaluated carefully before they are used. There is no

guarantee that the quality of test items in a published item bank is superior to that of test items that a skilled teacher can construct. The purpose of the test, relevant characteristics of the students to be tested, and the balance and emphasis of content as reflected on the teacher's test blueprint are the most important criteria for selecting test items. In addition, published test item banks seldom contain item analysis information such as difficulty and discrimination indices. However, this information can be calculated for each item that a teacher uses from a published item bank, and a teacher-made item file can be developed and maintained.

SUMMARY

After administering a test, the teacher must score it and interpret the results. In order to accurately interpret test scores, the teacher needs to analyze the performance of the test as a whole and of the individual test items. Information about how the test performed helps teachers to give feedback to students about test results and to improve test items for future use.

Scoring is the process of determining the first direct, uninterpreted measure of performance on a test, usually called the raw score. The raw score usually represents the number of right answers. Usually, test scores should not be converted to grades for the purpose of later computing a final average grade. Instead, the teacher should record actual test scores and then combine them into a composite score that can be converted to a final grade.

As a general rule, each objective-type test item should have equal weight. If knowledge of one concept is more important than knowledge of another concept, the teacher should sample the more important domain more heavily by writing more items in that area. Most machine-scoring systems assign one point to each correct answer; this seems reasonable for hand-scored tests as well.

A raw score sometimes is adjusted or corrected before it is interpreted. One procedure involves applying a formula intended to eliminate any advantage that a student might have gained by guessing correctly. Correcting for guessing is appropriate only when students have been instructed to not answer any item for which they are uncertain of the answer; students may interpret and follow this advice differently. Therefore the best approach is to advise all students to answer every item, and no correction for guessing should be applied.

Item analysis can be performed by hand or by the use of a computer program. Teachers should be familiar enough with the meaning of each item analysis statistic to correctly interpret the results. The difficulty index, ranging from 0 to 1.00, indicates the percentage of students who answered the item correctly. Items with p values of .20 and below are considered to be difficult, and those with p values of .80 and above are considered to be easy. However, interpretation of the difficulty index should take into account the quality of the instruction and the abilities of the students in that group. The discrimination index, ranging from -1.00 to + 1.00, is an indication of the extent to which the item was answered correctly more often by high-scoring students than by low-scoring students. In general, the higher the positive value, the better the test item; discrimination indices of .40 and higher indicate very good items. An item's ability to discriminate is highly related to its difficulty index. An item that is answered correctly by all students has a difficulty index of 1.00; the discrimination index for this item is 0.00, because there is no difference in performance on that item between high scorers and low scorers.

Flaws in test construction may have varying effects on students' scores, and therefore should be handled differently. If the correct answer to a multiple-choice item is inadvertently omitted from the test, no student will be able to answer the item correctly. In this case, the item simply should not be scored. If a flaw consists of a misspelled word in a true-false item that does not change the meaning of the statement, no adjustment should be made.

Teachers should develop a system for maintaining a pool or bank of items from which to select items for future tests. Item banks can be maintained in file boxes or drawers or on computer disks. Use of published test item banks should be based on the teacher's evaluation of the quality of the items as well as on the purpose for testing, relevant characteristics of the students, and the desired emphasis and balance of content as reflected in the teacher's test blueprint.

REFERENCES

Ebel, R. L., & Frisbie, D. A. (1991). *Essentials of educational measurement* (5th ed.). Englewood Cliffs, NJ: Prentice Hall.

Cangelosi, J. S. (1990). *Designing tests for evaluating student achievement*. New York: Longman.

Flynn, M. K., & Reese, J. L. (1988). Development and evaluation of classroom tests: A practical application. *Journal of Nursing Education, 27*, 61–65.

Jenkins, H. M., & Langley, C. G. (1991). A test protocol for large groups. *Nurse Educator, 16* (1), 8–10.

Mehrens, W. A., & Lehmann, I. J. (1991). *Measurement and evaluation in education and psychology* (4th ed.). Fort Worth, TX: Holt, Rinehart and Winston.

Nitko, A. J. (1996). *Educational assessment of students* (2nd ed.). Englewood Cliffs,

NJ: Prentice Hall.

Popham, W. J. (1990). *Modern educational assessment: A practitioner's perspective* (2nd ed.). Englewood Cliffs, NJ: Prentice Hall.

Waltz, C. F., Strickland, O. L., & Lenz, E. R. (1991). *Measurement in nursing research* (2nd ed.). Philadelphia: F. A. Davis.

10

Clinical Evaluation

Nursing, as a practice discipline, requires development of cognitive, affective, and psychomotor skills for the care of clients. Acquisition of knowledge alone is not sufficient; professional education includes a practice dimension, where students develop competencies for care of clients and learn to think and act like professionals. Through clinical evaluation the teacher arrives at judgments about the students' competencies in practice. In this chapter, concepts of clinical evaluation are explored; in chapter 11, specific clinical evaluation methods are presented.

It is through the students' clinical practice experiences that they develop a knowledge base for practice, cognitive abilities, professional values, and psychomotor and technological skills essential for delivering care. Clinical practice provides opportunities to apply concepts and theories to practice and to transfer learning from readings, class, and other experiences to care of clients. Clinical experiences are essential for higher level cognitive learning. Practice with real patients is not the same as simulations and other experiences with hypothetical client situations; it provides opportunity to deal with ambiguous client situations and unique cases not fitting the textbook picture, which require problem solving and critical thinking.

Schön (1990) emphasized the need for such learning in preparing for professional practice. Clinical experiences present problems and situations that do not lend themselves to resolution through application of theory and a technical rational approach. These problems may be difficult to identify, may present themselves as unique cases, and may be known by the professional but have no clear solutions (Schön, 1990). When faced with these uncertainties and unique client cases, students have an opportunity to develop their thinking and decision-making abilities to handle these situations.

Client situations in the swampy lowlands are contrasted from those in the high ground, represented by problems able to be solved by application of theory and research, a technical rational approach. Nursing students and nurses alike are faced with both of these types of problems. Through clinical practice students learn how to handle these situations and gain experience in solving varied client problems. They also develop the ability to initiate and respond to change, particularly important in today's health care system.

Other outcomes of clinical practice are learning to learn, to accept responsibility for one's own actions and decisions, and to think and act like a professional (Oermann, 1994a, 1994b; Reilly & Oermann, 1992). Professionals in any field are eternal learners through the duration of their careers. Continually expanding knowledge and changing needs of society influence nursing practice. While faculty attempt to prepare students for future practice, continued learning is essential as new knowledge and skills are introduced in the health fields and societal needs vary. In clinical practice students are faced with situations of which they are unsure; they are challenged to raise questions about care and practice and seek further learning. Students in clinical practice gain experience in identifying their own gaps in learning and how to meet these learning needs.

Clinical practice also enables students to accept responsibility for actions they take and their decisions about clients. They develop through their clinical experiences a sense of commitment to be responsible for their actions. This commitment has a cognitive component—an awareness of the need for accountability for actions and decisions related to practice—and a value dimension—accepting this responsibility in their own care of clients.

One other outcome of clinical practice is learning to think and act like a professional. In caring for clients and working with nurses and members of other disciplines, students gain an understanding of how professionals approach their clients' problems, how they interact with each other, and behaviors important in carrying out their roles in the practice setting. Through their observations of others in the role, they learn important role behaviors. In essence, they learn how to act like a professional in nursing through their observations of other professionals in the role (Oermann, 1997).

These outcomes of clinical practice are diagrammed in Figure 10.1. They provide a framework for faculty to use in evaluating students in the clinical setting, for they suggest outcomes of learning to be assessed in

Acquire knowledge, professional values, and psychomotor/technological skills for practice	Acquire problem-solving, decision-making, and critical-thinking abilities	Handle ambiguities; Initiate and respond to change
Learn how to learn	Accept responsibility and accountability	Think and act like a professional

Figure 10.1 Outcomes of clinical practice.

clinical practice. Not all outcomes are met in every course; for instance, some courses may not have technological skills to be acquired, but overall, most courses will move students toward achievement of these outcomes as they progress through the nursing program.

CONCEPT OF CLINICAL EVALUATION

Clinical evaluation is a process by which judgments are made about learners' competencies in practice. This practice may involve care of clients, other aspects of clinical practice, simulated experiences which students complete, and performance of varied skills and procedures. In all these dimensions of clinical evaluation, the teacher arrives at judgments about the students' competencies. Judgments influence the data collected, in essence, the observations made about students' performance. Deciding on the quality of performance and drawing inferences and conclusions from the data also involves judgments by the teacher. Clinical evaluation is not an objective process; it is subjective, involving judgments of the teacher as well as students and others involved in the process. Tanner (1994) cautioned faculty that no matter what model is used to guide clinical evaluation, "some degree of judgment will always be involved" (p. 243).

As discussed in chapter 1, the teacher's values influence evaluation. As such, it is important to be aware of values that may bias one's judgments of students. This is not to suggest that clinical evaluation may be value-free; the teacher's observations of performance and conclusions drawn will always be influenced by the teacher's values. The key is to develop an awareness of these values so as to avoid influencing clinical evaluation to a point of unfairness to the student. For instance, if the teacher prefers students who initiate discussions and participate actively in conferences, this value should not influence judgments about students' competencies in other areas. The teacher needs an awareness of this preference to avoid an unfair evaluation of other dimensions of clinical performance. Faculty should examine their own values, attitudes, and beliefs so they are aware of them as they teach and evaluate students in the clinical setting.

Clinical Evaluation vs. Grading

Clinical evaluation is not the same as grading. In evaluation, the teacher makes observations of performance and collects other types of data, then compares this information to a set of standards to arrive at a judgment. From this a quantitative symbol or grade may be applied to reflect the evaluation data and judgments made about performance. The clinical grade, such as pass–fail or A through F, is the quantitative symbol to represent the evaluation. Clinical performance may be evaluated and not graded, such as with formative evaluation; however, grades should not be assigned without sufficient evaluative data.

Norm- and Criterion-Referenced Clinical Evaluation

Clinical evaluation may be norm- or criterion-referenced as described in chapter 1. In norm-referenced evaluation, the student's clinical performance is compared with that of other students in the clinical group, indicating that the performance is better or worse than that of others in the group or that the student has more or less knowledge, skill, or ability than the other students. Rating students' clinical competencies in relation to others in the clinical group, for example, indicating that the student was "average," is a norm-referenced interpretation.

In contrast, criterion-referenced clinical evaluation involves comparing the student's clinical performance to predetermined criteria, and not to the performance of other students in the group. In this type of clinical evaluation, the criteria upon which to base performance are known in advance and used as the basis for evaluation. Indicating that the student has met the clinical objectives, or that performance reflects the criteria, regardless of how other students performed in the clinical setting, represents a criterion-referenced interpretation. In this system, the learner's position on a "performance continuum" is indicated in absolute terms, and not his or her rank within a group of learners (Ebel & Frisbie, 1991, p. 35).

Formative and Summative Clinical Evaluation

Clinical evaluation may be formative or summative. Formative evaluation in clinical practice provides feedback to learners about their progress in meeting the clinical objectives or developing competencies. The purposes of formative evaluation are to indicate areas where further learning is needed; enable students to develop their clinical knowledge, values, and skills further; and serve as a basis for additional instruction. Formative evaluation is, therefore, diagnostic in nature; with this type of evaluation, after identifying the learning needs, instruction is provided to move students forward in their learning. Considering that formative evaluation is diagnostic, it is not intended to be graded (Reilly & Oermann, 1992). Reviewing a student's assessment, for instance, for formative purposes would provide feedback on areas to be improved. Similarly, observing a student's initial performance of a skill in clinical practice, evaluating that performance, and giving feedback on it would serve a diagnostic purpose to improve subsequent performance. As such, these observations and judgments would not be graded.

Summative clinical evaluation, however, is designed for determining clinical grades, for it serves as a way of summarizing competencies the student has developed in clinical practice. Reilly and Oermann (1992) characterized summative evaluation as end-of-instruction evaluation, for it provides an assessment as to the extent to which the learner has achieved the clinical objectives or competencies at the end of a period of time, for example, at the end of the clinical course. Summative evaluation is not diagnostic; it is not intended to assist students in improving performance, nor to guide them in how to accomplish this. For much of clinical practice in a nursing program, summative evaluation comes too late for students to have an opportunity to improve performance. At the end of a course involving care of mothers and children, for instance, there may be many behaviors that the student would not have an opportunity to practice in subsequent courses.

Any protocol for clinical evaluation should include extensive formative evaluation and periodic summative evaluation. Formative evaluation is essential to provide feedback to improve performance while practice experiences are still available. A third type of clinical evaluation, confirmative, was described in chapter 1. Confirmative evaluation determines if learners have maintained their clinical competencies over time.

Fairness in Clinical Evaluation

Considering that clinical evaluation is not objective, the goal is to establish a fair evaluation system. Fairness involves three dimensions:

1. *Identifying the teacher's own values, attitudes, beliefs, and biases that may influence the evaluation process.* These may affect both the data collected about students and inferences made. In addition, students enter the

clinical setting with their own set of values, attitudes, beliefs, and biases that influence their self-evaluations of performance and responses to the teacher's evaluation and feedback. Students' acceptance of the teacher's guidance in clinical practice and information provided to them for improving performance is affected by each student's own value system. Developing a fair evaluation system, then, requires assessment by the teacher of his or her own values and acceptance of differences in how students respond to the evaluation process. In situations in which student responses inhibit learning, the teacher may need to intervene to guide students in more self-awareness of their own values and the effect of these values on learning.

2. *Basing clinical evaluation on predetermined objectives or competencies.* Clinical evaluation should be based on preset objectives or competencies to guide the evaluation process. Without these, neither teacher nor student has any basis for what to evaluate in clinical practice. What are the objectives of the clinical course or experiences to be met? What competencies is the student attempting to develop? These objectives or competencies provide a framework for faculty to use in observing performance and arriving at judgments about achievement in clinical practice. For instance, if the objectives of a clinical experience relate to developing communication skills, then the teacher's observations should be directed toward these skills, not toward other competencies unrelated to the experience.

3. *Developing a supportive clinical environment* in which students are free to learn, differences among students are accepted, and evaluation is viewed as a means of promoting growth of students, not controlling them. This climate for evaluation is important for students to seek guidance and accept feedback from the teacher, rather than avoiding the teacher in the clinical setting. Developing a supportive learning environment is also important because clinical practice is inherently stressful for students.

STRESS IN CLINICAL PRACTICE

There have been a number of studies in nursing education dealing with student stress and anxiety. Concern about making an error and harming the patient, limited knowledge and skills for practice, and difficulties in interacting with the teacher and others in the clinical setting are some of the stresses reported by students.

In an early study in this area, Pagana (1988) identified the stresses and threats experienced by students ($N=262$) in their first clinical experience in medical–surgical nursing courses. Using the Clinical Stress Questionnaire (CSQ), developed for the purpose of this research, Pagana reported that while students were stressed in clinical practice, a mean of 2.7 on a scale of 0 (none) to 4 (a great deal), they were significantly more challenged by these same experiences. The majority of students described feelings of inadequacy, feared they would harm the patient, were uncertain about some of their decisions, were frightened, and feared failing the clinical course. A number of students reported fear of the clinical teacher (n=68, 26%).

Other researchers also found that students were stressed in clinical practice in different courses and experiences (Beck & Srivastava, 1991; Kleehammer, Hart, & Keck, 1990; Reider & Riley-Giomariso, 1993; Williams, 1993; Wilson, 1994). Oermann (in press) compared the stresses in clinical practice between students (N=415) in associate degree (ADN) and baccalaureate (BSN) nursing programs. ADN students reported significantly higher stress in clinical practice than BSN students. The stress experienced by students increased as they progressed through the program; the semester prior to graduation was the most stressful time in terms of clinical practice for both groups of students. Stress was highest for students enrolled in pediatric nursing courses compared with other clinical courses (Oermann & Standfest, 1997).

The research suggests that clinical practice is inherently stressful for students, and teachers apparently may be one factor contributing to student stress (Kleehammer et al., 1990; Oermann, in press; Oermann, 1996; Pagana, 1988). This points to the need for teachers to be aware of the stressful nature of these learning experiences, to establish a supportive climate for learning in the clinical setting, to develop trusting relationships with students, and to be aware of their own behaviors and actions that may add to this stress.

The teacher should always remember that learning in the clinical setting is a *public event*. Students can not hide their lack of understanding or skill as they might in class. In clinical practice the possibility exists for many people to observe the student's performance—the teacher, client, peers, nursing staff, and other health providers. The nature of clinical learning, in and of itself, may create stress for learners in any health field.

FEEDBACK IN CLINICAL EVALUATION

Clinical evaluation, to be effective, needs to focus predominantly on providing feedback to the learner—formative evaluation—for without this feedback the student would receive limited guidance as to how to improve performance. Feedback is knowledge of results; it includes specific information about the student's performance to guide further practice and development of knowledge and skill. This feedback may be verbal, by describing observations and conclusions about performance followed by further instruction, and visual, by demonstrating correct performance. The ultimate goal is for students to progress to a point at which they judge their own performance, identify resources for their learning, and use those resources to develop competencies further.

Feedback provided by the teacher is augmented feedback, special cues from the teacher that direct the student's performance to improve it. Intrinsic feedback, internal to the student, represents the learner's own perceptions of performance and improvements needed in it. Once students have an underlying knowledge base and beginning skill, they can judge their own performance. Some students are more proficient than others in evaluating their performance in clinical practice and deciding how to modify it to reflect the predetermined criteria.

There are five principles for providing feedback to learners as part of the clinical evaluation process:

1. *Give precise and specific information to students*; general information about performance, such as "You need to work on your assessment," does not guide students in how to develop competencies further. Indicating instead the specific areas of data collection omitted and physical examination techniques that need improvement is more valuable to learners than a general description of their behavior.

2. For procedures and skills, *include both verbal and visual cues for students*, explaining the changes needed and demonstrating correct performance.

3. *Give feedback to students about their performance at the time of learning* or immediately following it. The longer the period of time between performance and feedback from the teacher, the less effective is the feedback. As time progresses, neither student nor teacher can remember specific areas of clinical practice to be improved.

4. *Adapt the feedback to the learner's needs*. Some students require more frequent and extensive feedback from the teacher than others. While the long-term goal is to develop self-reliant learners who can evaluate their own performance and make needed improvements, in beginning practice and with clinical situations that are new to learners, some students may require more frequent feedback.

5. Remember that *feedback is intended to be diagnostic*. After identifying areas in which further learning is needed, provide instruction and guidance for improving performance.

CLINICAL OBJECTIVES AND COMPETENCIES

There are different ways of specifying the outcomes to be achieved in clinical practice which in turn provide the basis for clinical evaluation. These may be developed in the form of clinical objectives or as competencies to be demonstrated in clinical practice. In general, these determine what is evaluated in clinical practice.

Clinical objectives represent the outcomes to be achieved in clinical practice. They may be separate objectives developed for a clinical course or represent the course objectives for which clinical practice is required for attainment (Reilly & Oermann, 1992). Regardless of the process used for their development, the clinical objectives reflect the outcomes of learning to be demonstrated and evaluated in clinical practice. The clinical objectives often address eight areas of learning:

1. Knowledge, concepts, and theories applicable to clinical practice;
2. Critical thinking within the context of clinical practice, including objectives related to assessment, diagnosis, planning, interventions, and evaluation of care;
3. Psychomotor and technological skills and other types of interventions;
4. Values related to care of clients;
5. Communication skills, ability to develop interpersonal relationships, and skill in collaboration;
6. Management of care, leadership abilities, and professional role;
7. Accountability and responsibility of the learner;
8. Self-development and continued learning.

Not all clinical courses will have objectives in each of these areas, and in some courses there may be other types of clinical objectives, such as those on research. This is a broad framework to guide teachers in developing clinical objectives. Sample clinical objectives are displayed in Table 10.1.

In some situations, the clinical objectives are generally stated, and therefore do not provide an adequate basis for evaluating students in clinical practice. In these instances, specific behaviors to be demonstrated in clinical practice may be identified. For example, the clinical objective "Use the nursing process in care of children and families" provides limited direction as to evaluating student attainment of it. More specific clinical behaviors may be developed to clarify the outcomes of learning to be evaluated, such as "Carries out a systematic assessment of children reflecting their developmental stage"; "Evaluates the impact of the health problem on the child and family"; and "Identifies resources for the family in coping

Table 10.1 Sample Clinical Objectives

Knowledge, concepts, and theories for clinical practice
- Uses principles of asepsis in caring for clients across settings.
- Applies family theories in care of mothers and children.
- Relates theories of pain to care of chronically ill children.

Critical thinking within context of clinical practice
- Collects significant data from multiple sources.
- Differentiates relevant from irrelevant data.
- Identifies alternate nursing diagnoses possible.
- Provides a sound rationale for decisions made about assessment data and diagnoses.
- Considers multiple nursing interventions and consequences of each.
- Develops outcome criteria for evaluating care of clients.

Psychomotor/technological skills and other interventions
- Is competent in performing physical examinations.
- Demonstrates skill in care of arterial lines.
- Performs competently the following procedures (list procedures and techniques to be evaluated as part of clinical course).

Values
- Accepts responsibility for assuring that clients have sufficient information for making informed decisions about care.
- Maintains confidentiality of patient information.
- Respects the inherent worth and dignity of clients.

Communication, interpersonal, and collaborative skills
- Identifies verbal and nonverbal techniques for communicating with clients.
- Develops interpersonal relationships with clients considering the demands and constraints of the health care system.
- Collaborates with other health providers in care of clients in varied community settings.

Management of care, leadership abilities, and professional role
- Analyzes the roles of the nurse in managed care.
- Demonstrates skill in delegating nursing activities to others.
- Coordinates care for clients in the clinic and other settings.

Accountability and responsibility
- Assumes responsibility for accessing needed resources for clients.
- Is accountable for responding to client concerns or working with others to resolve them.
- Completes clinical activities within planned time frame.

(continued)

Table 10.1 *(cont.)*

Self-development and responsibility for continued learning
- Identifies own clinical learning needs.
- Uses resources for learning to improve clinical performance.
- Seeks guidance as needed for carrying out procedures and care of clients.

---

with the child's health problem and managing care at home," to cite a few examples.

Competencies are the abilities to be demonstrated by the learner in clinical practice. For nurses in practice, these competencies reflect the proficiencies needed to perform a particular task or carry out their defined role in the health care setting. Competencies for nurses are assessed as part of their initial employment and orientation to the health care setting and on an ongoing basis. Snyder-Halpern and Buczkowski (1990) described a performance-based approach to staff development to evaluate nurses' clinical competencies. Three distinct phases are included in this approach. In the first phase, post-hire, nurses participate in a performance-based assessment designed to evaluate competencies to meet "designated performance expectations as specified in employee job descriptions" (p. 8). In phase II, specific instruction is provided to remedy deficiencies and enable nurses to demonstrate performance suitable for their own jobs. In the third phase, there is ongoing assessment of each nurse's performance to validate clinical competencies and move them toward developing expertise in clinical practice.

For each of the competencies identified for clinical practice, there are typically performance criteria established for determining achievement of the competency. Table 10.2 provides an example of a competency with related performance criteria. These criteria are important in clinical evaluation, for they provide objective and measurable criteria for determining competent performance.

Caution must be exercised in developing clinical objectives, specific behaviors, and competencies to avoid having too many for evaluation, considering the number of learners for whom the teacher is responsible, the types of clinical experiences available, and time allotted for clinical practice. In addition, they should reflect more general learning outcomes and not be too specific. Highly specific objectives and competencies create difficulties in planning learning experiences for students and collecting sufficient data for arriving at judgments about students' performance. Regardless of how the evaluation system is developed, the clinical

Table 10.2 Sample Competency and Performance Criteria

Competency: IV injection of medications

Performance criteria:
- ❏ Checks physician's order.
- ❏ Checks that medication is for IV use.
- ❏ Determines proper method for administering IV medication.
- ❏ Assembles appropriate equipment.
- ❏ Uses correct diluent.
- ❏ Mixes IV medication in proper concentration.
- ❏ Identifies patient correctly.
- ❏ Explains procedure to patient.
- ❏ Positions patient according to method IV medication will be administered.
- ❏ Selects appropriate vein (if applicable).
- ❏ Cleans site.
- ❏ Administers medication at proper rate.
- ❏ Flushes tubing.
- ❏ Documents IV medication correctly on flow sheet.

objectives and competencies need to be realistic and useful for guiding the evaluation.

SUMMARY

Through clinical evaluation, the teacher arrives at judgments about students' performance in clinical practice. These judgments influence the data collected, in essence, the observations made about students' performance, and the inferences and conclusions drawn from the data. Clinical evaluation, therefore, is not an objective process; it is subjective, involving judgments of the teacher as well as students and others involved in it. In designing an evaluation system for clinical practice, the teacher bases the evaluation on the clinical objectives or competencies. These provide the framework for learning in clinical practice and basis for evaluating performance. The performance of students is judged in relation to these objectives or competencies.

Although a framework such as this is essential in clinical evaluation, teachers also need to examine their own beliefs about the evaluation process and purposes it serves in nursing. Clarifying their own values, beliefs, attitudes, and biases that may affect evaluation is an important first step. It is also important to recognize the inherent stress of clincal practice for many students and develop a supportive learning environment. Other concepts of evaluation, presented initially in chapter 1, were re-examined in terms of evaluating performance in the clinical setting. Specific methods for carrying out this evaluation are described in the next chapter.

REFERENCES

Beck, D. L., & Srivastava, R. (1991). Perceived level and sources of stress in baccalaureate nursing students. *Journal of Nursing Education, 30,* 127–133.

Ebel, R. L., & Frisbie, D. A. (1991) *Essentials of educational measurement* (5th ed.). Englewood Cliffs, NJ: Prentice Hall.

Kleehammer, K., Hart, A. L., & Keck, J. F. (1990). Nursing students' perceptions of anxiety-producing situations in the clinical setting. *Journal of Nursing Education, 29,* 183–187.

Oermann, M. H. (1994a). Professional nursing education in the future: Changes and challenges. *JOGNN, 5,* 153–159.

Oermann, M. H. (1994b). Reforming nursing education for future practice. *Journal of Nursing Education, 33,* 215–219.

Oermann, M. H. (1996). Research on teaching in the clinical setting. In K. R. Stevens (Ed.), *Review of research in nursing education* (Vol. VII, pp. 91–126). New York: National League for Nursing.

Oermann, M. H. (1997). *Professional nursing practice.* Norwalk, CT: Appleton & Lange.

Oermann, M. H. (In press). Differences in clinical experience of ADN and BSN students. *Journal of Nursing Education.*

Oermann, M. H., & Standfest, K. A. (1997). Differences in stress and challenge in clinical practice among ADN and BSN students in varying clinical courses. *Journal of Nursing Education, 36,* 228–233..

Pagana, K. D. (1988). Stresses and threats reported by baccalaureate students in relation to an initial clinical experience. *Journal of Nursing Education, 27,* 418–424.

Reider, J. A., & Riley-Giomariso, O. (1993). Baccalaureate nursing students' perspectives of their clinical nursing leadership experience. *Journal of Nursing Education, 32,* 127–132.

Reilly, D. E., & Oermann, M. H. (1992). *Clinical teaching in nursing education.* New York: National League for Nursing.

Schön, D. A. (1990). *Educating the reflective practitioner.* San Francisco: Jossey-Bass.

Snyder-Halpern, R., & Buczkowski, E. (1990). Performance-based staff development. *Journal of Nursing Staff Development, 6,* 7–11, 24.

Tanner, C. A. (1994). Professional judgment in evaluation. *Journal of Nursing Education, 33,* 243–244.

Williams, R. P. (1993). The concerns of beginning nursing students. *Nursing &
    Health Care, 14,* 178–184.
Wilson, M. E. (1994). Nursing student perspective of learning in a clinical setting.
    Journal of Nursing Education, 33, 81–86.

11

Clinical Evaluation Methods

After establishing a framework for evaluating students in clinical practice and exploring values and beliefs that may influence evaluation, the teacher identifies a variety of methods or strategies for collecting data on student performance in clinical practice and arriving at judgments about it. Evaluation methods, or strategies, are the actual techniques used for assessing learning in clinical practice. There are many evaluation methods available for use in nursing programs. Some methods, such as games and simulations, are more appropriate for formative evaluation, whereas others are useful for either formative or summative evaluation. In this chapter, varied methods for evaluating clinical practice are presented.

SELECTION OF CLINICAL EVALUATION METHODS

There are several factors to consider in selecting evaluation methods for clinical practice. First, select evaluation methods that provide information on how well students are meeting or have met the clinical objectives or competencies. The evaluation methods used in a clinical course, or for selected clinical experiences, should provide data on achievement of the objectives or performance of designated competencies. For many clinical objectives there are multiple strategies that would be appropriate, thereby allowing flexibility in choosing methods for evaluation.

Most evaluation methods provide data on multiple clinical objectives. For example, a short written assignment in which students compare two different data sets might relate to objectives on critical thinking, writing, and patient assessment. In deciding on evaluation methods, the teacher reviews the clinical objectives and selects methods that provide information on achievement of multiple objectives or competencies.

Second, vary the clinical evaluation methods. Considering the different clinical evaluation strategies available, the teacher has a wealth of methods from which to choose. Varying the methods maintains student interest and reflects individual needs, abilities, and characteristics of learners. Some students may be more proficient in methods that depend on writing, while others prefer strategies such as conferences and other discussions. Planning for multiple evaluation methods in clinical practice as long as these are congruent with the outcomes to be evaluated reflects these differences among students. It also avoids relying on one method, such as rating scales, for determining the entire clinical grade.

Third, select evaluation methods that are realistic considering the nature of the clinical experience, resources available, and constraints. Planning for an evaluation method that depends on clients with specific health problems or status, unique family situations, and other particular circumstances may not be realistic considering the varied types of clinical experiences of students in the course. Some methods require resources for implementation, for example, space for discussion and equipment for simulated experiences. If these resources are not available in the clinical settings in which students have experiences, then other strategies should be considered. Some games, for instance, require a certain number of participants, thereby restricting their use.

Fourth, differentiate methods intended for formative versus summative evaluation and clarify this for students. Some of the strategies designed for clinical evaluation are strictly to provide feedback to students on areas for improvement and are not graded. As described in the previous chapter, students need prompt feedback accompanied by suggestions for improvement and remedial instruction. Other methods, though, such as rating forms and certain written assignments, may be used for summative purposes and therefore computed as part of the clinical grade.

Fifth, review the purpose and number required of each assignment completed by students in clinical practice. What are the purposes of these assignments, and how many are needed to demonstrate competency? In some clinical courses, students complete an excessive number of assignments, such as care plans. How many such assignments, regardless of whether they are for formative or summative purposes, are needed to develop an understanding of the care-planning process? Students benefit mainly from continuous feedback from the teacher, not from repetitive assignments that contribute little to their development of clinical knowledge and skills. Vary the clinical assignments, give prompt feedback, and when students have demonstrated competency, allow them to progress to other more stimulating activities.

Sixth, in deciding on clinical evaluation methods, consider faculty time for completing the evaluation, providing feedback, and grading. Some of the clinical assignments, for instance, may be completed in conferences or by groups of students, rather than as individual activities, and evaluated by the teacher at that time.

CLINICAL EVALUATION METHODS

The rest of the chapter presents clinical evaluation methods for use in nursing education programs. Some of these methods were examined in earlier chapters, since they are also applicable to testing situations and use in the classroom and other types of educational settings.

Observation

The predominant strategy for evaluating clinical performance is observing the performance of students in clinical practice and other settings. Although observation is widely used, there are threats to its validity and reliability. First, observations of students may be influenced by the teacher's values, attitudes, and biases, as discussed in the previous chapter. There also may be overreliance on first impressions that might change with further observations of the student (Nitko, 1996). This points to the need for a series of observations before drawing conclusions about performance.

Second, in observing performance in the clinical setting in particular, there are many aspects of the performance on which the teacher may focus attention. For instance, in observing a student administer an IV medication, the teacher may focus mainly on the technique used for its administration, ask limited questions about the purpose of the medication, and make no observations of how the student interacts with the client and documents its administration. Another teacher observing this same student may focus on these other aspects. The same situation, therefore, may yield somewhat different observations.

Third, the teacher may arrive at incorrect judgments about the observations, such as inferring that a student is inattentive during conference when in fact the student is thinking about the comments made by others in the group. It is important that the teacher discusses observations with students, obtains their perceptions of behavior, and is willing to modify his or her own inferences when new data are presented.

Fourth, every observation in the clinical setting reflects only a sampling, or window, of the learner's performance during a clinical experience. An observation of the same student at another point in time may reveal a different level of performance. The same holds true for observations of the teacher; on some clinical days, and for some classes, the teacher's behaviors do not represent a typical level of performance. An observation of the same teacher during another clinical experience and class may reveal a different quality of teaching.

These are important concepts in making observations of students. Once again, they point to the need for a series of observations of clinical performance in varied situations, and having multiple sources of data before drawing conclusions about students' competencies. Bott (1996) emphasized the need to base those observations on predetermined objectives or competencies and "have clearly in mind what is to be observed" (p. 189). The objectives or competencies assist the teacher in keeping the observation focused to the learning outcomes. This is not to indicate, however, that other aspects of performance are insignificant; the teacher should make observations of student performance beyond those suggested by the objectives or competencies. These are particularly important for providing feedback to students in the clinical setting.

If the teacher finds that limited experiences, with patients, through simulations, and with other methods, are available for evaluating students' clinical performance, then the objectives or competencies may need revision to be more broadly stated, applicable to a wider range of experiences, and fewer in number. This is particularly true considering the shift of clinical practice for students to community-based systems.

ANECDOTAL NOTES

There are several ways of recording observations of students in the clinical setting, learning laboratory, and other settings: anecdotal notes, checklists, and rating scales. These are summarized in Table 11.1.

Anecdotal notes are narrative descriptions of observations made of students. They provide a means of recording the observations made of learners in clinical practice. Nitko (1996) indicated that anecdotal notes were particularly appropriate for naturally occurring performances.

Anecdotal notes may include only a description of the observations or may also reflect the teacher's interpretations or conclusions about the performance. Considering the issues raised with observations, the teacher should discuss those recorded in anecdotal notes with students and be willing to incorporate the students' own judgments about performance in the evaluation. Reviewed frequently with students, anecdotal notes are

Table 11.1 Methods for Recording Observations

Anecdotal notes	Used for recording descriptions of observations made of students in the clinical setting; may also include interpretations or conclusions about the performance
Checklists	Used primarily for recording observations of procedures and techniques performed by students; includes steps for carrying out the procedures and also may include errors in performance to check
Rating scales	Used for recording judgments about students' performance in clinical practice. Includes a set of defined clinical objectives, behaviors, or competencies and scale for rating the degree of competence (graduated scale or pass–fail)

useful for giving feedback to learners and gathering their own perceptions of their performance. While they may be used for summative evaluation, they are most appropriate for formative evaluation.

CHECKLISTS

A checklist is a list of specific behaviors or activities to be observed, with a place for checking whether or not they were present during performance (Nitko, 1996, p. 270). A checklist often lists steps to be followed in performing a procedure or technique. Some checklists also include inappropriate steps and errors in performance, as well as the correct steps in sequence. Nitko (1996) suggested that specifying possible errors on the checklist promoted their review with students and focused remedial instruction on these errors in performance. Checklists facilitate students' self-evaluation of performance; students can review and evaluate their

Table 11.2 Sample Checklist

Student Name _____

Instructions to teacher/examiner: Observe the student performing the following procedure and check the steps completed properly by the student. Check only those steps that the student performed properly. After completing the checklist, discuss performance with the student, reviewing aspects of the procedure to be improved.

IV Injection of Medication

Checklist:

❑ Checks physician's order.

❑ Checks that medication is for IV use and states this if asked by teacher/examiner.

❑ States proper method for administering the IV medication.

❑ Assembles appropriate equipment.

❑ Uses correct diluent.

❑ Mixes IV medication in proper concentration.

❑ Cleans site properly.

❑ Administers medication at correct rate.

❑ Flushes tubing.

❑ Documents IV medication correctly on flow sheet.

---

own performance prior to assessment by the teacher.

Linn and Gronlund (1995) identified four steps for designing checklists:

1. List clearly each step in the procedure students should follow.
2. Add to the list specific errors students often make in the procedure.
3. Sequence the steps in proper order including where errors might occur.
4. Develop the list into a form that allows checking off the steps as they are performed in the proper sequence.

In designing checklists, avoid specifying every possible step in the procedure, resulting in cumbersome lists of steps, and focus instead on critical ones and where they fit in the sequence. For procedures and techniques for which there are multiple ways of performing them, allow for this flexibility in developing the checklist. Specify critical steps and indicate examples of alternate ways of carrying them out. Table 11.2 provides an example of a checklist developed from the sample competency and performance criteria in Table 10.2.

RATING SCALES

Rating scales provide a means of recording judgments about observed performance of students in clinical practice. A rating scale contains two parts: (a) a set of clinical objectives, behaviors, or competencies the student is to demonstrate in clinical practice and therefore provide the basis for observation, and (b) a scale for rating the students' performance of those objectives, behaviors, or competencies.

Rating scales are most useful for summative evaluation of performance; after observing students over a period of time, the teacher draws conclusions about performance, rating it according to the scale provided with the instrument. These scales also may be used to evaluate specific activities students complete in clinical practice, for instance, rating a student's presentation of a clinical conference or quality of teaching provided to a client. Other uses of rating scales are to: (a) help students focus their attention on critical behaviors to be performed, (b) give specific feedback to students about the strengths and weaknesses of their performance, and (c) demonstrate student growth in clinical competencies over a designated time period if the same rating scale is used (Nitko, 1996, p. 272).

There are many varieties of rating scales used for clinical practice. The scales may be multidimensional, with descriptors such as:

- Letters: A, B, C, D, E or A, B, C, D, F;
- Numbers: 1, 2, 3, 4, 5;
- Qualitative labels: Excellent, very good, good, fair, and poor; Exceptional, above average, average, and below average;
- Frequency labels: Always, usually, frequently, sometimes, and never;
- Other labels such as: Independent, supervised, assisted, marginal, and dependent (Bondy, 1983; Tower & Majewski, 1987).

A short description included with these letters, numbers, and labels for each of the objectives, behaviors, and competencies rated improves objectivity and consistency (Nitko, 1996). An example is found in Figure 11.1.

Or, scales may be two-dimensional, such as pass–fail and satisfactory–unsatisfactory. Karns and Nowotny (1991) reported that the majority ($n=80$, 59%) of BSN nursing programs in their survey used pass-fail for rating clinical performance rather than a multidimensional system. Both types of scales, however, are appropriate for clinical evaluation.

Objective: Collects relevant data from client

Exceptional	Above-Average	Average	Below-Average
Differentiates relevant from irrelevant data; analyzes multiple sources of data; establishes complete data base; identifies data needed for evaluating all possible nursing diagnoses	Collects significant data from clients; uses multiple sources of data as part of assessment; identifies possible nursing diagnoses based on data	Collects significant data from clients; uses data to develop nursing diagnoses	Does not collect significant data and misses important cues in data; unable to explain relevance of data for nursing diagnoses

Figure 11.1 Sample rating scale.

A main difficulty in using rating scales is apparent by a review of the typical scale descriptors. What are the differences between "Excellent" and "Very good?" Between "Above Average" and "Average?" Between a "1" and "2?" Is there consensus among teachers using the rating scale as to what constitutes these levels of performance for each objective, behavior, and competency evaluated? This problem even exists when descriptions are provided for each of the levels of the rating scale, such as in the previous example. Teachers may differ in their judgments of whether the student collected *relevant* data, if *multiple* sources of data were used, if the database was *complete* or not, if *all possible* nursing diagnoses were considered, and so forth. Scales based on frequency labels are often difficult to implement because of limited experiences for students to practice and demonstrate a level of skill "always, usually, frequently, sometimes, and never." How should faculty rate students' performance in situations in which they practiced the skill perhaps once or twice in the clinical setting? Even with two-dimensional scales, such as pass-fail, there is room for variability among faculty because of judgment entering into the observation and conclusions drawn.

Nitko (1996, p. 277) identified common errors that occur with rating scales applicable to their use in rating clinical performance:

1. *Leniency error* results when the teacher tends to rate all students toward the high end of the scale. This also occurs with teachers who give higher ratings to students they like.

2. *Severity error* is the opposite of leniency error, tending to rate all students toward the low end of the scale.

3. *Central tendency error* is hesitancy to mark either end of the rating scale and use of the middle part of the scale only. Rating students only at the extremes or middle of the scale limits validity of the ratings for all students and does not distinguish one student's performance from the others, making the ratings unreliable.

4. *Halo effect* is a judgment based on a general impression of the student. With this error the teacher lets an overall impression influence the ratings of specific dimensions and aspects of performance. The teacher places a "halo" around the student that affects ability to evaluate and rate specific objectives, behaviors, and competencies. This halo may be positive, giving a higher rating than the student deserves, or negative, letting a general negative impression of the student result in lower ratings of specify aspects of performance.

5. *Personal bias* occurs when the teacher's biases influence ratings, for example, favoring nursing students who do not work while attending school over ones who are employed.

6. *Logical error* results when similar ratings are given for items on the scale that are logically related to one another. This is a problem with some rating scales in nursing. For instance, there may be multiple behaviors on communication skills to be rated; while the teacher has observed some of these behaviors, the same rating is given to all behaviors on communication. It may be that some of the behaviors in the rating scale can be combined.

To avoid some of these difficulties with rating scales,

1. *Be alert to the possible influence of one's own values, attitudes, and beliefs* in observing performance and drawing conclusions about it.

2. *Use the clinical objectives, behaviors, or competencies* as a way of focusing observations in the clinical setting. Give students feedback on other observations made about their performance.

3. *Collect sufficient data on student performance* before drawing conclusions about it. It is important to observe the student more than one time before rating performance. Rating scales used for clinical practice generally represent a summary of the observations made about students' performance.

4. *Make a series of observations* over a period of time and in varied clinical situations. If this is not possible, develop additional strategies for evaluation so that performance is evaluated with different methods and at different points in time.

5. *Do not rely on first impressions*; they may not be correct.

6. *Discuss observations with students*, obtain their perceptions of behavior, and be willing to modify judgments and ratings when new data are presented.

7. *Review the clinical experiences* and ask if they provide sufficient data for completing the rating scale. Other experiences might be needed, either

with clients or simulated experiences. Or, the clinical objectives or competencies might need to be modified to be more realistic considering the clinical teaching circumstances.

8. *Avoid using rating scales as the only source of data* about a student's performance; use multiple evaluation methods for clinical practice.

9. *Rate each objective, behavior, or competency* individually based on the observations made of performance and conclusions drawn. Do not rate all students high, low, or in the middle; similarly, do not let your general impression of the student or personal biases influence rating.

10. Do not rate items for which data are not available or for which conclusions are not possible regarding the student's level of performance; leave these blank.

11. If the rating form is ineffective for judging student performance, then revise and re-evaluate it. Is the instrument valid, reliable, and easy to use, as described in chapter 2?

Although there are difficulties with using rating scales, they are, nevertheless, an important clinical evaluation method, for they allow teachers to rate performance over time and note patterns of performance. There are many different types of rating scales used for evaluating clinical performance in nursing programs. Sample forms are included in Appendix A.

Simulations

A simulation creates an experience that represents reality. Hanna (1991) described a major advantage of simulation as providing experience for students without the constraints of a real-life situation. Simulations present situations requiring problem solving, decision making, and critical thinking, fostering development of cognitive skills and enabling students to reflect on their own thinking without the demands of clinical practice.

They may be presented in paper-and-pencil format; incorporate multimedia, such as videotapes and interactive video that combines computer simulation with videotapes; involve computer simulations; and use various other materials to portray the reality of a situation. Video and other types of media clips may be used to present the scenario for analysis, portraying it more clearly than in a paper-and-pencil format. Label videotapes used for teaching that present brief scenarios which may then be used for evaluating ability to identify problems, consider solutions, arrive at decisions, and critique the thinking of others. With a computer simulation, the computer defines the situation for problem solving and decision making and may provide feedback to the students on their solutions. With some simulations, students act out roles and perform certain actions to accompany their decision making. The simulation may incorporate models for evaluating certain skills and procedures, mannequins, and simulated patients.

In some simulations, introductory information is presented to the learner for decision making; data then are added to the situation altering the decisions and expanding the scenario for further analysis. This type of simulation provides practice for learners in decision making and feedback on the process used for arriving at decisions.

Simulations are most appropriate for formative evaluation, providing feedback from teacher and peers. They allow learners to experience a situation and gain an awareness of their feelings, perceptions, and responses before facing or encountering the situation in the clinical setting.

Simulations, however, also may be developed for summative evaluation. Bramble (1994) described the Objective Structured Clinical Assessment (OSCA) to evaluate clinical competencies. In this method, two types of stations are set up, clinical and static. Clinical stations assess the student's ability to take a patient's history and perform a limited physical examination while being observed by an examiner and scored on performance. Specific criteria are used for rating performance. At static stations, students answer test items, multiple-choice or short-answer, based on the previous station. Bramble suggested that one benefit of the OSCA is that clinical skills to be evaluated are divided into their various components and are judged based on predetermined performance standards. Simulated patients, trained to enact the role, are used to maintain objectivity; they are instructed to present certain patient data in the history, mimic physical findings, and portray the same scenario for each student. Varied adaptations of the OSCA may be used for evaluation of clinical performance.

Games

Games are contests played with rules, goals, and certain activities to perform for the purpose of learning (Reilly & Oermann, 1992). While games such as crossword puzzles, trivia questions, and board games, to name a few, may be used for clinical evaluation, they are appropriate only for formative evaluation. Their role in evaluation is to give immediate feedback to participants (Fuszard, 1995).

Media Clips

As indicated earlier, simulations may be developed in many different formats, one of which incorporates multimedia. Media clips, short segments of a videotape, a film, an interactive video, and other forms of media, may be viewed by students as a basis for discussions in clinical conferences, written assignments, group activities, and other types of experiences. Media clips often are more effective than descriptions of a clinical situation in paper-and-pencil format and in a discussion because they allow the student to see and hear the client. Keep the segment viewed by students short so that they can focus on critical aspects of it as related to the outcomes to be evaluated. Media clips are appropriate for assessing students' ability to apply concepts and theories to the client situation depicted in the media clip, identify problems and multiple approaches possible, arrive at decisions and explore their consequences, and engage in critical thinking. Although the assignments students complete after viewing the media may be graded, media clips are most valuable for formative evaluation, particularly in a group format in which students can discuss their ideas and receive feedback from the teacher and peers.

Written Assignments

Written assignments accompanying the clinical experience are effective strategies for evaluating students' problem solving, decision making and critical thinking, as discussed in chapter 7; understanding of content relevant to clinical practice; and ability to express ideas in writing. Evaluation of written assignments was described in chapter 6. There are many types of written assignments appropriate for clinical evaluation, although research is limited in this area (Oermann, 1996).

Nursing care plans from the practice setting or with a format developed by the teacher enable the student to analyze the client's health problems and plan realistic care considering the constraints within the health care system. In using care plans for clinical evaluation, students should be moved quickly into the format of the health care agency, rather than having long detailed care plans designed for learning purposes that may not be relevant to actual practice. Modifying standardized care plans for individual clients and generating and modifying computerized care plans from a nursing information system are important skills to be evaluated with this type of assignment (Brown & Kellum, 1997).

Case study and *case method* were described in chapter 7. These are effective strategies for evaluating problem solving, decision making, and critical thinking. They may be developed around actual clients for whom the students have cared or around hypothetical case situations related to the clinical objectives. Although these assignments may be completed as individual activities, they also are appropriate for group work, in clinical conferences, or as required assignments outside of clinical practice time, and may be presented for group discussion in conferences. Analysis of case studies and shorter descriptions of clinical situations, in the case method format, may be evaluated for formative purposes or as part of the grade for clinical practice. Varied types of case methods were described in chapter 7 and therefore are not repeated in this chapter.

Process recording provides a way of evaluating students' abilities to analyze interactions they have had with clients or through simulated experiences. Process recordings are useful for providing feedback to students about their interactional skills, but the analysis of the communication also may be graded.

Journals provide an opportunity for students to document their responses to clinical experiences. An important outcome of clinical journals is to enable students to "think aloud," recording their perceptions of the clinical experiences (Brown & Sorrell, 1993). The purpose of the journal is not to develop scholarly writing skills, but instead to provide an avenue for expressing feelings and engaging in a dialogue with teachers about them. Callister (1993) described journals as a way of reflecting on feelings and attitudes and documenting the cognitive development of learners throughout a clinical course.

Hodges (1996) developed this perspective further in her conceptualization of journal writing. She proposed a leveling of journal-writing reflecting progression in cognitive development, as well as other outcomes. In this model, there are four levels for journal-writing, beginning with summarizing, describing, and reacting to clinical experiences and progressing toward analyzing and critiquing positions, issues, and views of others. Although typically journals provide an opportunity for giving feedback to learners and are not graded, Hodges (1996) proposed grading journals based on grammar, spelling, sentence structure, clarity, logical flow of argument, and substantive critical thought (p. 140). Other experts, however, do not recommend grading journals as they often reflect the feelings, perceptions, and responses of learners.

Brown and Sorell (1993) suggested these guidelines for clinical journals:

1. Identify outcomes for using the journal and the goals to be attained, such as documenting observations of patients, critiquing data according to relevant theories, suggesting hypotheses, and evaluating them.

2. Provide clear guidelines for journal entries, for instance, having students write their own learning objectives and how they are meeting them; write a summary of a clinical event or an article relevant to clinical practice; and select a practice issue and write a focused argument as to the position taken.

3. Provide thoughtful and immediate feedback to students to develop a dialogue between teacher and student (pp. 17–18).

Sedlak (1992, 1997) examined the use of journals for beginning nursing students. Students documented their responses to clinical practice in them; qualitative analysis by Sedlak indicated that the journals enabled students to reflect on their clinical experiences, promoted communication between teacher and students, and documented student learning and development of critical thinking skills in clinical practice.

Short papers for evaluating critical thinking and other cognitive skills were described in chapter 7. These are important clinical evaluation methods, considering the emphasis in nursing programs on development of these skills and the need to document their achievement. In addition, whereas many of the clinical evaluation methods are better suited for formative evaluation—providing feedback to students—papers developed around clinical practice may be evaluated for grading purposes. Examples of papers students might complete are:

- Compare different sets of client data. What are similarities in the data? Differences? How do these influence decisions about patient problems?
- Compare health problems of different individuals, families, and communities and propose solutions for them.
- Given a client problem, identify alternate perspectives possible.
- Design alternate approaches possible for varied health problems, discuss the consequences of each, and specify outcome criteria for their evaluation.
- Consider multiple approaches that could be used in a clinical situation, state which approach the student would use, and provide a rationale for this decision.
- Identify a decision made in clinical practice involving clients and staff and present evidence on which their reasoning was based.
- Analyze conclusions drawn about a client, evidence to support these conclusions, and alternate ones possible given the same evidence.
- Analyze an issue in clinical practice, alternate courses of actions that could be used, and why each one would be effective.
- Identify a problem or an issue students faced in their clinical practice, critique the approaches they used for resolving it, and identify alternate approaches that might have been used.
- Given an issue involving clients, nurses, other health providers, and health care in general, analyze different points of view, perspectives, and positions.
- Take a position about an issue in clinical practice and present an argument to support their position.

Term papers also may be completed about clinical practice, providing an opportunity for students to critique relevant literature, summarize their ideas, and demonstrate the use of theories and concepts for analyzing clinical problems. Term papers enable teachers to judge writing ability of students. Along this same line, a series of drafts of these papers, combined with prompt feedback on writing, promote development of writing skill among students.

Other written assignments, such as teaching plans and documentation of client care, also provide another source of evaluation data for clinical practice. Guidelines for evaluating written assignments were presented in chapter 6 and therefore are not repeated here. In planning the clinical evaluation protocol, however, exercise caution in the type and number of written assignments so they promote learning without unnecessary repetition.

Portfolio Assessment

A student portfolio documents meaningful projects that take place in clinical practice over a period of time. Bott (1996) described portfolios as collections of projects students engaged in for significant periods of time that resulted in products demonstrating their learning (p. 190). Portfolio assessment has a "tremendous potential for both evaluation and promotion of learning" (Forker & McDonald, 1996, p. 6). Portfolios may be developed over time, varied abilities may be documented in the portfolio and then evaluated based on predetermined criteria, and students may assess their own performance and development. Portfolios are valuable for clinical evaluation in that students provide evidence in their portfolios to confirm their clinical competence and document new learning resulting from their clinical experiences. Forker and McDonald (1996) recommended portfolios for validating community-based competencies, as faculty often supervise students at a distance and in a variety of community agencies.

In addition to assessment, portfolios are used as teaching tools, for professional development of teachers, and for research (Mitchell, 1992). The contents of the portfolio depend on the purpose it is to serve in evaluation. Nitko (1996) differentiated two types of portfolios: best work and growth-and-learning progress. Best-work portfolios include evaluation portfolios in which the contents of the portfolio provide evidence that the student has demonstrated certain competencies and achievements in clinical practice; these are appropriate for summative clinical evaluation. Growth-and-learning-progress portfolios are designed for monitoring students' progress and self-reflection of learning outcomes at several points in time. These contain products and work of the students in process, at the intermediate stages, for the teacher to review and provide feedback (Nitko, 1996.)

For clinical evaluation, these purposes may be combined. The portfolio may be developed initially for growth and learning, with products and entries reviewed periodically by teachers for formative evaluation, and then as a best-work portfolio with completed products providing evidence of clinical competencies. The best-work portfolio may then be graded.

The content of the portfolio depends on the clinical objectives and outcomes to be achieved with it. The portfolio may include evidence of student learning for a series of clinical experiences, over the duration of a clinical course, or for documenting competence in terms of curriculum or program outcomes. Most portfolios serve more than one purpose and set of outcomes; these need to be clearly identified as the basis for determining the contents of the portfolio.

Multiple types of documentation may be included in the portfolio, depending on the objectives to be evaluated with it, such as entries similar to a journal, short papers students have completed, term papers, reports of group work, reports and analyses of observations made in the clinical setting, self-reflections of clinical experiences, and other products students complete associated with clinical practice that demonstrate their learning and development of competencies. The decision as to content to include in the portfolio depends on

1. its purpose—is the portfolio for demonstrating growth and learning in clinical practice, is it a best-work portfolio, or will it combine these purposes? and
2. specific objectives or outcomes to be evaluated through the documentation in the portfolio.

There are several steps to follow in setting up a portfolio system for clinical evaluation. These were developed from the work of Nitko (1996, pp. 281–282).

Step 1: Identify the purposes of the portfolio.

• Will the portfolio serve as a means of assessing students' development of clinical competencies, focusing predominantly on the growth of students? Will the portfolio provide evidence of students' best work in clinical practice, including products reflecting their learning over a period of time? Or will the portfolio meet both demands, enabling the teacher to give continual feedback to students on the process of learning and projects on which they are working, as well as providing evidence of their accomplishments and achievements in clinical practice?

• Will the portfolio be used for formative or summative evaluation?

Or both?

• Will the portfolio provide evaluation data for use in a clinical course, or for curriculum- and program-evaluation purposes?

• Will the portfolio serve as a means of assessing prior learning, and therefore have an impact on the types of learning experiences or courses that students complete; for instance, for assessing the prior learning of RNs entering a baccalaureate or higher degree program or for licensed practical nurses entering an associate degree program?

• What is the role of students, if any, in defining the focus and content of the portfolio?

Step 2: Identify the type of content to be included in the portfolio.

• What types of entries are required in the portfolio, for example, products developed by students, descriptions of projects with which students are involved, descriptions of clinical learning experiences and reactions to them, observations made in clinical practice and analysis of them, and papers completed by students, among other types of information needed to achieve the purposes of the portfolio?

• In addition to required entries, what other types of content and entries might be included in the portfolio?

• Who determines the content of the portfolio and types of entries? Teacher only? Student only? Both?

• Will the entries be the same for all students or individualized by the student?

• What is the minimum number of entries to be considered satisfactory?

• How should the entries in the portfolio be organized, or will students organize it themselves?

• What is the time frame for each entry to be included in the portfolio, and at what points in time should it be submitted to faculty for review and feedback?

• Will teacher and student meet in a conference for discussion of the portfolio?

Step 3: Decide on the evaluation of the portfolio entries including criteria for evaluation of individual entries and the portfolio overall.

• How will the portfolio be integrated within the clinical evaluation grade and course grade, if at all?

• What criteria will be used to evaluate, and perhaps score, each type of entry and the portfolio as a whole?

• Will only the teacher evaluate the portfolio and its entries? Or will students evaluate their own progress and work? Or will the evaluation be a collaborative effort?

These steps and questions to be answered provide guidelines for teachers in developing a portfolio system for clinical evaluation in a course or for other purposes in the nursing program.

Conferences

Ability to present ideas orally is an important outcome of clinical practice. Sharing information about a client, leading others in discussions about clinical practice, presenting ideas in a group format, and giving lectures and other types of speeches are important skills to be developed. Working with other disciplines requires the ability to communicate effectively with them, as well as with clients and their families. Directions for the future suggest that this ability will be even more important, as nursing practice takes place increasingly in community-based systems in which collaboration is needed with many individuals and groups. Conferences provide a method for developing oral communication skills and for evaluating competency in this area. Other uses of conferences, as related to evaluation of problem-solving, decision-making, and critical-thinking skills, and how to conduct discussions that stimulate higher level learning were described in chapter 7.

There are many types of conferences appropriate for clinical evaluation depending on the objectives to be met: (a) clinical conferences, discussions about clients' care and other aspects of practice; (b) post-conferences at the conclusion of a clinical experience; (c) issue conferences involving group discussion of issues associated with clinical practice, professional issues, and cultural, social, economic, and political issues (Reilly & Oermann, 1992, p. 407); (d) interdisciplinary conferences; and (e) critical incident conferences in which details of significant incidents in practice are explored by the group (Brookfield, 1995).

Criteria for evaluating conferences include the ability to:

- Present ideas clearly and in a logical sequence to the group;
- Participate actively in the group discussion;
- Offer ideas relevant to the topic under discussion;
- Demonstrate knowledge of the content discussed in the conference;
- Assume a leadership role, if relevant, in promoting group discussion and arriving at group decisions;
- Lead the group, if relevant, in identifying problems to be solved and evaluating different approaches possible; arriving at decisions based on sound reasoning; and critiquing evidence used as a basis for decisions; and
- Contribute multiple perspectives to the discussion.

Clinical Examination

Clinical examinations are structured evaluations of clinical performance outside of the clinical setting for the purpose of summative evaluation. Clinical examinations provide for greater control over the environment in which practice occurs, limiting the effect of distractions on performance. Clinical examinations, however, should be balanced with observations in clinical practice to assess the abilities of students to transfer learning to the practice setting and function effectively within the reality of different clinical environments.

Clinical examinations, since they are intended for summative evaluation, are typically used at the completion of a clinical course or set of clinical experiences for assessing multiple objectives. They include several clinical evaluation methods, such as viewing videotapes, participating in simulations, completing related written assignments, and demonstrating procedures and skills that are observed and evaluated by the teacher or an examiner. Frequently students are given clinical scenarios related to the course content but involving novel situations that the students have not yet explored. After analyzing the scenario, students may complete several activities, such as completing an assessment, deriving nursing diagnoses, developing plans, specifying interventions, and indicating how care would be evaluated. Questions for critical thinking may be easily integrated within these types of activities. Students may be asked to demonstrate skills, on a model or with simulated patients, that are observed and evaluated by the teacher or examiner. Any type of activity relevant to the clinical objectives and able to be carried out in a simulated setting may be incorporated into the examination. Clinical examinations are useful for evaluating clinical knowledge and performance for courses in which the teacher is not readily available for observing actual care of clients.

In some clinical examinations, the student's performance is videotaped for rating at a later time by more than one teacher or examiner; multiple ratings are then available for grading purposes. Graf (1993) also recommended videotaping performance of skills for formative purposes because it provides for prompt feedback to students, lowers stress associated with having skills observed by the teacher, and saves faculty time.

In setting up the clinical examination, identify objectives or outcomes to be evaluated, skills to be performed as part of the examination, and how the examination will be structured. For evaluation of skills, checklists or rating scales may be used; other evaluation methods depend on the type of activities that students complete in the examination.

Self-Evaluation

Development of the ability to evaluate own learning and competency is another important outcome of a nursing program (Oermann, 1994). Self-evaluation begins with the first clinical experience and develops throughout the student's nursing program, continuing into professional practice. Self-evaluation serves four purposes:

1. to discuss students' clinical performance and obtain their perceptions of their competencies;
2. to identify strengths and areas for future learning from the teacher's and student's perspectives;
3. to provide feedback to students and identify additional learning experiences needed for improving performance; and
4. to enhance communication between teacher and student.

Self-evaluation is appropriate only for formative evaluation, and as such should not be graded.

SUMMARY

This chapter built on the concepts of clinical evaluation examined in chapter 10. Multiple clinical evaluation methods are available for assessing student competencies in clinical practice. There are several factors to consider in selecting these evaluation methods. First, evaluation methods should provide information on how well students are meeting or have met the clinical objectives or competencies. The evaluation methods used in a clinical course, or for selected clinical experiences, should provide data on achievement of the objectives or performance of designated competencies. For many clinical objectives, there are multiple appropriate strategies, thereby allowing flexibility in choosing methods for evaluation.

Clinical evaluation methods should be realistic considering the nature of the clinical experience, resources available, and constraints of the clinical teaching situation. The teacher should decide if the evaluation strategy is intended for formative or summative evaluation. Some of the strategies designed for clinical evaluation are strictly to provide feedback to students on areas for improvement and are not graded. As described in the previous chapter, students need prompt feedback on their clinical performance, accompanied by suggestions for improvement and remedial instruction. Other methods, though, such as rating forms and certain written assignments, may be used for summative purposes and therefore may be computed as part of the clinical grade.

In deciding on clinical evaluation methods, consider the purpose and number required of assignments completed in clinical practice and faculty time for evaluating them, providing feedback, and grading them. Some of the clinical assignments, for instance, may be completed in conferences or by groups of students, rather than as individual activities, and evaluated by the teacher at that time.

The predominant strategy for evaluating clinical performance is observing the performance of students in clinical practice and other settings. Although observation is widely used, there are threats to its validity and reliability. Observations of students may be influenced by the teacher's values, attitudes, and biases, as discussed in the previous chapter. There also may be overreliance on first impressions that might change with further observations of the student.

In observing performance in the clinical setting, there are many aspects of the performance on which the teacher may focus attention. Every observation reflects only a sampling, or window, of the learner's performance during a clinical experience. An observation of the same student at another point in time may reveal a different level of performance. These issues in observing clinical performance point to the need for a series of observations before drawing conclusions about performance. It is equally important for the teacher to discuss observations with students, obtain their perceptions of behavior, and be willing to modify the teacher's own inferences when new data are presented.

There are several ways of recording observations of students in the clinical setting, learning laboratory, and other settings: anecdotal notes, checklists, and rating scales. These were described in the chapter. Common errors that occur with rating scales applicable to their use in rating clinical performance also were described.

A simulation creates an experience that represents reality. A major advantage of simulation is that it provides experience for students without the constraints of a real-life situation. Simulations present situations requiring problem solving, decision making, and critical thinking, fostering development of cognitive skills and enabling students to reflect on their own thinking without the demands of clinical practice. Often multimedia are integrated in the simulation; other forms of media clips also may be used for clinical evaluation.

Written assignments accompanying the clinical experience are effective strategies for evaluating students' problem solving, decision making and critical thinking, as discussed in chapter 7; understanding of content relevant to clinical practice; and ability to express ideas in writing. There are many types of written assignments appropriate for clinical evaluation.

A student portfolio documents a meaningful project or collections of projects that students worked on in clinical practice over a period of time. Varied abilities may be documented in the portfolio and then evaluated based on predetermined criteria, and students may assess their own performance and development. Portfolios are valuable for clinical evaluation in that students provide evidence in their portfolios to confirm their clinical competencies and document new learning resulting from their clinical experiences.

Other clinical evaluation methods are conference, clinical examination, and self-evaluation. The evaluation methods presented in this chapter provide the teacher with a wealth of strategies from which to choose in evaluating students' clinical performance.

REFERENCES

Bondy, K. N. (1984). Clinical evaluation of student performance: The effects of criteria on accuracy and reliability. *Research in Nursing and Health, 7*, 25–33.

Bott, P. A. (1996). *Testing and assessment in occupational and technical education*. Boston: Allyn and Bacon.

Bramble, K. (1994). Nurse practitioner education: Enhancing performance through the use of the Objective Structured Clinical Assessment. *Journal of Nursing Education, 33*, 59–65.

Brookfield, S. D. (1995). *Becoming a critically reflective teacher*. San Francisco: Jossey-Bass.

Brown, H. N., & Sorrell, J. M. (1993). Use of clinical journals to enhance critical thinking. *Nurse Educator, 18* (5), 16–19.

Brown, P. A., & Kellum, S. S. (1997). Computers in nursing practice. In M. H. Oermann (Ed.), *Professional nursing practice* (pp. 189–212). Norwalk, CT: Appleton & Lange.

Callister, L. C. (1993). The use of student journals in nursing education: Making meaning out of clinical experience. *Journal of Nursing Education, 32*, 185–186.

Forker, J. E., & McDonald, M. E. (1996). Methodologic trends in healthcare professions: Portfolio assessment. *Nurse Educator, 21* (5), 9–10.

Fuszard, B. (1995). Gaming. In B. Fuszard (Ed.), *Innovative teaching strategies in nursing* (2nd ed., pp. 112–120). Gaithersburg, MD: Aspen.

Graf, M. A. (1993). Video taping return demonstrations. *Nurse Educator, 18* (4), 29.

Hanna, D. R. (1991). Using simulations to teach clinical nursing. *Nurse Educator, 16* (2), 28–31.

Hodges, H. F. (1996). Journal writing as a mode of thinking for RN-BSN students: A leveled approach to learning to listen to self and others. *Journal of Nursing Education, 35*, 137–141.

Karns, P., & Nowotny, M. (1991). Clinical structure and evaluation in baccalaureate schools of nursing. *Journal of Nursing Education, 30*, 207–210.

Linn, R. L., & Gronlund, N. E. (1995). *Measurement and assessment in teaching* (7th ed.). Englewood Cliffs, NJ: Prentice Hall.

Mitchell, R. (1992). *Testing for learning*. New York: The Free Press.

Nitko, A. J. (1996). *Educational assessment of students* (2nd ed.). Englewood Cliffs, NJ: Prentice Hall.

Oermann, M. H. (1994). Professional nursing education in the future: Changes and challenges. *JOGNN, 23*, 153–159.

Oermann, M. H. (1996). Research on teaching in the clinical setting. In K. R. Stevens (Ed.). *Review of research in nursing education* (Vol. VII, pp. 91–126). New York: National League for Nursing.

Reilly, D. E., & Oermann, M. H. (1992). *Clinical teaching in nursing education*. New York: National League for Nursing.

Sedlak, C. A. (1992). Use of clinical logs by beginning nursing students and faculty to identify learning needs. *Journal of Nursing Education, 33*, 389–394.

Sedlak, C. A. (1997). Critical thinking of beginning baccalaureate nursing students during the first clinical nursing course. *Journal of Nursing Education, 36*, 11–18.

Tower, B. L., & Majewski, T. V. (1987). Behaviorally based clinical evaluation. *Journal of Nursing Education, 26*, 120–123.

12

Interpreting Test Scores

A s a measurement technique, a test results in a score—a number. As discussed in chapter 1, a number has no intrinsic meaning; it must be compared with something that has meaning in order to interpret it. A test score, therefore, must be interpreted in order to be meaningful and useful for decision making (Ebel & Frisbie, 1991). Whether these interpretations are norm-referenced or criterion-referenced, a basic knowledge of statistical concepts is necessary to assess the quality of teacher-made or published tests, understand standardized test scores, summarize assessment results, and explain test scores to others.

TEST SCORE DISTRIBUTIONS

Some information about how the test performed as a measurement instrument can be obtained from computer-generated test and item analysis reports. In addition to providing item analysis data such as difficulty and discrimination indexes, such reports often summarize characteristics of the score distribution. If the teacher does not have access to machine scoring and computer software for test and item analysis, many of these analyses can be done by hand, albeit more slowly.

When a test is scored, the teacher is left with a collection of raw scores. Often these scores are recorded according to the names of students, in alphabetical order. As an example, suppose that the scores displayed in Table 12.1 resulted from the administration of a 65-point test to 16 nursing students.

Table 12.1 List of Students in a Class and Their Raw Scores on a 65-Point Test

Student	Score	Student	Score
A. Allen	53	I. Ignatius	48
B. Brown	54	J. Jimanez	55
C. Chen	52	K. Kelly	52
D. Dunlap	52	L. Lynch	42
E. Edwards	54	M. Meyer	47
F. Finley	57	N. Nardozzi	60
G. Gunther	54	O. O'Malley	55
H. Hernandez	56	P. Purdy	53

Glancing at this group of numbers, the teacher would find it difficult to answer such questions as (Nitko, 1996, p. 449):

1. Are the scores widely scattered or grouped together?
2. Did any individuals score much higher or much lower than the majority of students?
3. What was the range of scores obtained by the majority of students?
4. Did a majority of students obtain high or low scores on the test?

To make them easier to visualize, the scores should be arranged in an orderly way, usually from highest to lowest, as in Table 12.2. Ordering the scores in this way makes it obvious that the scores ranged from 42 to 60, and that one student's score was much lower than those of other students. But the teacher still cannot visualize easily how a typical student performed on the test or the general characteristics of the obtained scores. Removing student names, listing each score once, and tallying how many times each score occurs results in a frequency distribution, as in Table 12.3. By displaying scores in this way, the score obtained by any individual student becomes less important than the general nature of the scores made by the group (Lyman, 1991).

The frequency distribution also can be represented graphically as a histogram. In Figure 12.1, the scores are ordered from lowest to highest along a horizontal line, left to right, and the number of asterisks above each score indicate the frequencies. Frequencies also can be indicated on a histogram by bars, with the height of each bar representing the frequency of the corresponding score, as in Figure 12.2.

A frequency polygon is another way to display a score distribution graphically. A dot is made above each score value to indicate the frequency

Table 12.2 Rank Order of Students From Table 12.1 with Raw Scores Ordered from Highest to Lowest

Student	Score	Student	Score
N. Nardozzi	60	A. Allen	53
F. Finley	57	P. Purdy	53
H. Hernandez	56	C. Chen	52
J. Jimanez	55	K. Kelly	52
O. O'Malley	55	D. Dunlap	52
B. Brown	54	I. Ignatius	48
E. Edwards	54	M. Meyer	47
G. Gunther	54	L. Lynch	42

Table 12.3 Frequency Distribution of Raw Scores from Table 12.1

Raw score	Frequency
61	0
60	1
59	0
58	0
57	1
56	1
55	2
54	3
53	2
52	3
51	0
50	0
49	0
48	1
47	1
46	0
45	0
44	0
43	0
42	1
41	0

with which that score occurred; if no one obtained a particular score, the dot is made on the baseline, at zero. The dots then are connected with straight lines to form a polygon or curve. With a small number of scores,

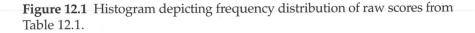

```
                              *         *
                          *   *    *   *
*                     *   *   *   *   *   *   *           *
41 42 43 44 45 46 47 48 49 50 51 52 53 54 55 56 57 58 59 60 61
```

Figure 12.1 Histogram depicting frequency distribution of raw scores from Table 12.1.

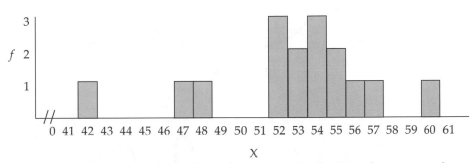

Figure 12.2 Bar graph depicting frequency distribution of raw scores from Table 12.1.

Note: X = scores; f = frequencies.

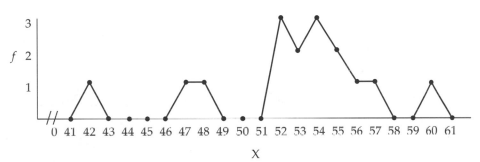

Figure 12.3 Frequency polygon depicting frequency distribution of raw score from Table 12.1.

Note: X = scores; f = frequencies.

the shape of the curve often is uneven or irregular; with a larger number of scores, the curve would take on a smoother, more regular shape (Mehrens & Lehmann, 1991). Figure 12.3 shows a frequency polygon based on the histogram in Figure 12.1. Histograms and frequency polygons thus show general characteristics such as the range of scores, shape of the

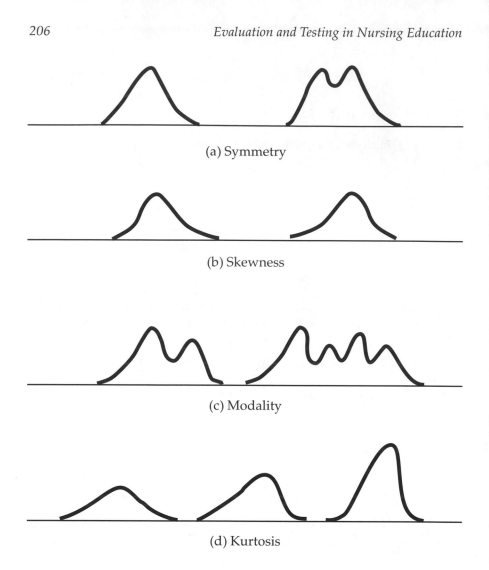

Figure 12.4 Characteristics of a score distribution.

From R. L. Ebel and D. A. Frisbie (1991), *Essentials of Educational Measurement* (5th ed., p. 58). Englewood Cliffs, NJ: Prentice Hall. Copyright 1991 by Prentice Hall. Reprinted with permission.

distribution, and most frequently obtained scores (Lyman, 1991).

The characteristics of a score distribution can be described on the basis of its symmetry, skewness, modality, and kurtosis. These characteristics are illustrated in Figure 12.4. A symmetric distribution or curve is one in which there are two equal halves; the halves are mirror images of each other. Nonsymmetric or asymmetric curves have a cluster of scores or peak at one end and a tail extending toward the other end. This type of curve is said to be skewed; the direction in which the tail extends indicates whether the distribution is positively or negatively skewed. The tail of a positively skewed curve extends toward the right, in the direction of positive numbers on a scale, and the tail of a negatively skewed curve extends toward the left, in the direction of negative numbers. A positively skewed distribution thus has the largest cluster of scores at the low end of the distribution, which seems counterintuitive. The distribution of test scores from Table 12.1 is nonsymmetric and negatively skewed. Remember that the lowest possible score on the test was 0 and the highest possible score was 65; the scores were clustered between 43 and 60.

Frequency polygons and histograms can differ in the number of peaks they contain; this characteristic is called modality, referring to the mode or the most frequently occurring score in the distribution. If a curve has one peak, it is unimodal; if it contains two peaks, it is bimodal. A curve with many peaks is multimodal. The peaks of bimodal and multimodal distributions do not have to be exactly of equal height (Lyman, 1991, p. 53). The relative flatness or peakedness of the curve is referred to as kurtosis. Flat curves are described as platykurtic, moderate curves are said to be mesokurtic, and sharply peaked curves are referred to as leptokurtic (Ebel & Frisbie, 1991). The histogram depicted in Figure 12.1 is a bimodal, platykurtic distribution.

The shape of a score distribution depends on characteristics of the test as well as the abilities of the students who were tested (Nitko, 1996). Some teachers make grading decisions as if all test score distributions resembled a normal curve, that is, they attempt to "curve" the grades. An understanding of the characteristics of a normal curve would dispel this notion. A normal distribution is a bell-shaped curve that is symmetric, unimodal, and mesokurtic. Figure 12.5 illustrates a normal distribution.

Many human attributes such as height, weight, and intelligence appear to be distributed according to this shape, with the largest number of persons in the middle range with respect to any of these characteristics (Polit, 1996). However, most score distributions obtained from teacher-made tests do not approximate a normal distribution. This is true for several reasons. The characteristics of a test greatly influence the resulting score distribution; a very difficult test tends to yield a positively skewed curve. Likewise, the abilities of the students influence the test score distribution. Regardless of the distribution of the attribute of intelligence among the human population, this characteristic is not likely to be distributed normally among a class of nursing students or a group of newly hired registered nurses

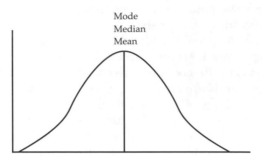

Figure 12.5 The normal distribution.

(RNs). Because admission and hiring decisions tend to select those individuals who are most likely to succeed in the nursing program or job, a distribution of IQ scores from a class of 16 nursing students or 16 newly hired RNs would tend to be negatively skewed. Likewise, knowledge of nursing content is not likely to be normally distributed, since those who have been admitted to a nursing program or hired as staff nurses cannot be said to be representative of the population in general. Therefore, grading procedures that attempt to apply the characteristics of the normal curve to a test score distribution are likely to result in unwise and unfair decisions.

Measures of Central Tendency

One of the questions to be answered when interpreting test scores is "What score is most characteristic or typical of this distribution?" A typical score is likely to be in the middle of a distribution, with the other scores clustered around it. Therefore, an index of central tendency is used to indicate this score value (Polit, 1996). Three measures of central tendency commonly used to interpret test scores are the mode, median, and mean.

As was previously discussed, the mode is the most frequently occurring score in the distribution; it must be a score actually obtained by a student. It can be identified easily from a frequency distribution or graphic display without mathematical calculation. As such, it provides a rough indication of central tendency. The mode, however, is the least stable measure of central tendency because it tends to fluctuate considerably from one sample to another drawn from the same population (Polit, 1996). That is, if the same 65-item test that yielded the scores in Table 12.1 was administered to a different group of 16 nursing students in the same school who had taken the same course, the mode might differ considerably. In addition, as in the distribution depicted in Figure 12.1, the mode has two or more values in some distributions, making it difficult to specify one typical score. A uniform distribution of scores has no mode; such distributions are likely to be obtained when the number of students is small, the range of scores is large, and each score is obtained by only one student.

The median, sometimes abbreviated Mdn, is the point that divides the distribution of scores into equal halves. It is a value above which fall 50% of the scores and below which fall 50% of the scores; thus it represents the 50th percentile. The median does not have to be an actual obtained score. In an even number of scores, the median is located halfway between the two middle scores; in an odd number of scores, the median is the middle score. Because the median is an index of location, it is not influenced by the value of each score in the distribution. Thus, it is usually a good indication of a typical score in a skewed distribution containing extreme high or low scores (Nitko, 1996).

The mean often is referred to as the "average" score in a distribution, reflecting the mathematical calculation that determines this measure of central tendency. It is usually abbreviated as M or $\bar{X}$. The mean is computed by summing each individual score and dividing by the total number of scores, as in the following formula:

$$M = \frac{\Sigma X}{N} \qquad \text{[Equation 12.1]}$$

where M is the mean, ΣX is the sum of the individual scores, and N is the total number of scores (Polit, 1996, p. 47). Thus, the value of the mean is affected by every score in the distribution. This property makes it the preferred index of central tendency when a measure of the total distribution is desired. However, the mean is sensitive to the influence of extremely high or low scores in the distribution, and as such, it may not reflect the typical performance of a group of students (Nitko, 1996, p. 454).

There is a relationship between the shape of a score distribution and the relative locations of these measures of central tendency. In a normal distribution, the mean, median, and mode have the same value, as shown in Figure 12.5. In a positively skewed distribution, the mean will yield the highest measure of central tendency and the mode will give the lowest; in a negatively skewed distribution, the mode will be the highest value and the mean the lowest. Figure 12.6 depicts the relative positions of the three measures of central tendency in skewed distributions.

The mean of the distribution of scores from Table 12.1 is 52.75; the

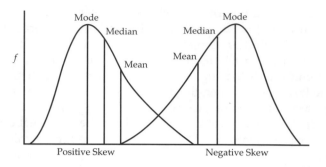

Figure 12.6 Measures of central tendency in skewed distributions. From D. F. Polit (1996). *Data Analysis and Statistics for Nursing Research,* p. 50. Stamford, CT: Appleton & Lange. Copyright 1996 by Appleton & Lange. Reprinted with permission.

median is 53.5. The fact that the median is slightly higher than the mean confirms that the median is an index of location or position and is insensitive to the actual score values in the distribution. The mean, since it is affected by every score in the distribution, was influenced by the one extreme low score. Because the shape of this score distribution was negatively skewed, it is expected that the median would be higher than the mean, since the mean is always pulled in the direction of the tail (Polit, 1996, pp. 47–50).

Measures of Variability

It is possible for two score distributions to have similar measures of central tendency and yet be very different. The scores in one distribution may be tightly clustered around the mean, and in the other distribution, the scores may be widely dispersed over a range of values. Measures of variability are used to determine how similar or different the students are with respect to their scores on a test.

The simplest measure of variability is the range, the difference between the highest and lowest scores in the distribution. For the test score distribution in Table 12.3, the range is 18 (60 - 42 = 18). The range is sometimes expressed as the highest and lowest scores, rather than a difference score. Because the range is based on only two values, it can be highly unstable. The range also tends to increase with sample size; that is, test scores from a large group of students are likely to be scattered over a wide range because of the likelihood that an extreme score will be obtained (Polit, 1996, p. 51).

The standard deviation, usually abbreviated as *SD* or *s*, is the most common and useful measure of variability. Like the mean, it takes into consideration every score in the distribution. The standard deviation is based on differences between each score and the mean. Thus, it characterizes the average amount by which the scores differ from the mean. The standard deviation is calculated in four steps:

1. Subtract the mean from each score $(X - M)$ to compute a deviation score (x), which can be positive or negative.
2. Square each deviation score (x^2), which eliminates any negative values. Sum all of the squared deviation scores $(\Sigma\, x^2)$.
3. Divide this sum by the number of test scores to yield the variance.
4. Calculate the square root of the variance.

Although other formulas can be used to calculate the standard deviation, the following definitional formula represents these four steps:

$$SD = \sqrt{\frac{\Sigma\, x^2}{N}}$$ [Equation 12.2]

where SD is the standard deviation, Σx^2 is the sum of the squared deviation scores, and N is the number of scores (Ebel & Frisbie, 1991, p. 61; Polit, 1996, p. 53).

The standard deviation of the distribution of scores from Table 12.1 is 4.1. What does that value mean? A standard deviation of 4.1 represents the average deviation of scores from the mean. On a 65-point test, 4 points is not a large average difference in scores. If the scores cluster tightly around the mean, the standard deviation will be a relatively small number; if they are widely scattered over a large range of scores, the standard deviation will be a larger number (Ebel & Frisbie, 1991).

INTERPRETING AN INDIVIDUAL SCORE

Interpreting the Results of Teacher-Made Tests

The ability to interpret the characteristics of a distribution of scores will assist the teacher to make norm-referenced interpretations of the meaning of any individual score in that distribution. For example, how should the teacher interpret P. Purdy's score of 53 on the test whose results were summarized in Table 12.1? With a median of 53.5, a mean of 52.75 and a standard deviation of 4.1, a score of 53 is about "average." All scores between 49 and 57 fall within one standard deviation of the mean, and thus are not significantly different from one another. On the other hand,

N. Nardozzi can rejoice because a score of 60 is almost two standard deviations higher than the mean; thus, this score represents achievement that is much better than that of others in the group. The teacher should probably plan to counsel L. Lynch, because a score of 42 is more than two standard deviations below the mean, much lower than others in the group.

Some teachers need to make criterion-referenced interpretations of individual test scores. A student's score on the test is compared to a preset standard or criterion, and the scores of other students are not considered. The percentage-correct score is a derived score that is often used to report the results of tests that are intended for criterion-referenced interpretation. The percentage correct is a comparison of a student's score with the maximum possible score; it is calculated by dividing the raw score by the total number of items on the test. Although many teachers believe that percentage-correct scores are an objective indication of how much students really know about a subject, in fact, these scores can change significantly with the difficulty of the test items. Since percentage-correct scores are often used as a basis for assigning letter grades according to a predetermined grading system, it is important to recognize that they are determined more by test difficulty than by true quality of performance. Consequently, teachers may need to adjust raw scores before calculating percentage-correct scores when it is evident that the test was much more difficult than the teacher expected or desired (Lyman, 1991, pp. 92–94).

The percentage-correct score should not be confused with percentile rank, often used to report the results of standardized tests. The percentile rank describes the student's relative standing within a group and therefore is a norm-referenced interpretation. The percentile rank of a given raw score is the percentage of scores in the distribution that occur at or below that score. A percentile rank of 83, therefore, means that the student's score is equal to or higher than the scores made by 83% of the students in that group; one cannot assume that the student answered 83% of the test items correctly. Because there are 99 points that divide a distribution into 100 groups of equal size, the highest percentile rank that can be obtained is the 99th. The median is at the 50th percentile. Differences between percentile ranks mean more at the highest and lowest extremes than they do near the median (Ebel & Frisbie, 1991; Lyman, 1991).

Interpreting the Results of Standardized Tests

The results of standardized tests usually are intended to be used to make norm-referenced interpretations. Before making such interpretations, the teacher should keep in mind that standardized tests are more relevant to general rather than specific instructional goals. Additionally, the results of standardized tests are more appropriate for evaluations of groups than of individuals. Consequently, standardized test scores should not be used to determine grades for a specific course or to make a decision to hire, promote, or terminate an employee. Like most educational measures, standardized tests provide gross, not precise, data about achievement. Therefore, results should be interpreted with the understanding that only large differences in scores indicate real differences in achievement levels (Cangelosi, 1990).

Standardized test results usually are reported in derived scores such as percentile ranks, standard scores, and norm-group scores. Because all of these derived scores should be interpreted in a norm-referenced way, it is important to specify an appropriate norm group for comparison. The standardized test manual typically presents norm tables in which each raw score is matched with an equivalent derived score. Standardized test manuals may contain a number of norm tables; the norm group on which each table is based should be fully described. The teacher should take care to select the norm group that most closely matches the composition of the group whose scores will be compared to it (Lyman, 1991). For example, when interpreting the results of National League for Nursing comprehensive tests, the performance of a group of baccalaureate nursing students should be compared with a norm group of baccalaureate nursing students. Norm tables sometimes permit finer distinctions such as size of program, geographical region, and public vs. private affiliation.

SUMMARY

In order to be meaningful and useful for decision making, test scores must be interpreted in norm-referenced or criterion-referenced ways. Knowledge of basic statistical concepts is necessary to make valid interpretations and to explain test scores to others.

Scoring a test results in a collection of numbers known as raw scores. To make raw scores understandable, they can be arranged in frequency distributions or displayed graphically as histograms or frequency polygons. Score distribution characteristics such as symmetry, skewness, modality, and kurtosis can assist the teacher in understanding how the test performed as a measurement tool, as well as to interpret any one score in the distribution.

Measures of central tendency and variability also aid in interpreting individual scores. Measures of central tendency include the mode, median, and mean; each measure has advantages and disadvantages for use. In a normal distribution, these three measures will coincide. Most score distributions from teacher-made tests do not meet the assumptions of a normal curve. The shape of the distribution can determine the most appropriate index of central tendency to use. Variability in a distribution can be described roughly as the range of scores or more precisely as the standard deviation.

Teachers can make criterion-referenced or norm-referenced interpretations about individual student scores. Norm-referenced interpretations of any individual score should take into account the characteristics of the score distribution, some index of central tendency, and some index of variability. The teacher thus can use the mean and standard deviation to make judgments about how an individual student's score compares with those of others.

A percentage-correct score is calculated by dividing the raw score by the total possible score; thus it compares the student's score to a preset standard or criterion and does not take the scores of other students into consideration. A percentage-correct score is not an objective indication of how much a student really knows about a subject because it is affected by the difficulty of the test items. The percentage-correct score should not be confused with percentile rank, which describes the student's relative standing within a group and therefore is a norm-referenced interpretation. The percentile rank of a given raw score is the percentage of scores in the distribution that occur at or below that score.

The results of standardized tests usually are reported as percentile ranks or other norm-referenced scores. Teachers should be cautious when interpreting standardized test results so that comparisons with the appropriate norm group are made. Standardized test scores should not be used to determine grades or to make personnel decisions, and results should be interpreted with the understanding that only large differences in scores indicate real differences in achievement levels.

REFERENCES

Cangelosi, J. S. (1990). *Designing tests for evaluating student achievement*. New York: Longman.

Ebel, R. L., & Frisbie, D. A. (1991). *Essentials of educational measurement* (5th ed.). Englewood Cliffs, NJ: Prentice Hall.

Lyman, H. B. (1991). *Test scores and what they mean*. Englewood Cliffs, NJ: Prentice Hall.

Mehrens, W. A., & Lehmann, I. J. (1991). *Measurement and evaluation in education and psychology* (4th ed.). Fort Worth, TX: Holt, Rinehart and Winston.

Nitko, A. J. (1996). *Educational assessment of students* (2nd ed.). Englewood Cliffs, NJ: Prentice Hall.

Polit, D. F. (1996). *Data analysis & statistics for nursing research*. Stamford, CT: Appleton & Lange.

13

Grading

E valuating students in the classroom and clinical practice provides the basis for assigning a grade to represent their achievement. Grades may be given for individual assignments students complete, for quizzes, tests, and other learning activities, and for the course as a whole. The grade is a symbol reflecting the achievement of students. This chapter examines uses of grades in nursing programs, problems with grading, grading frameworks, and how to compute grades for nursing courses.

PURPOSES OF GRADES

In preceding chapters there was extensive discussion about formative and summative evaluation. Through formative evaluation, the teacher provides feedback to the learner on a continuous basis. In contrast, summative evaluation is conducted periodically, to indicate the student's achievement at the end of the course or a point in time within the course. Summative evaluation provides the basis for arriving at grades in the course. Grading, or marking, is defined as the use of symbols, for instance, the letters A through F, to report student achievement. It is the process of assigning a symbol to represent the quality of the student's performance. Grading is used for summative purposes, indicating through the use of symbols how well the student met the course and clinical objectives.

Grades need to be based on careful evaluation practices, valid and reliable test results, and multiple evaluation measures. No grade should be determined on one evaluation method or one assignment completed by students; grades reflect instead a combination of various tests and other evaluation methods. Along a similar line, there may be many activities students complete that are not included in their grade. Not all of the students' achievements in a course are incorporated into the grade. A focus on formative evaluation in nursing courses results in many of these activities being evaluated by the teacher but not graded.

Although some would argue about the many problems associated with grading, particularly in clinical practice, grades have numerous uses in nursing education programs. Grades serve three broad purposes: (a) instructional, (b) administrative, and (c) guidance and counseling. Grades for instructional purposes indicate the achievement of students in the course, a measurement of *what* students have learned and their competencies at the end of the course or point in time within it. Ebel and Frisbie (1991) suggested that grades are an important means of stimulating, directing, and then rewarding the educational efforts of students.

The second purpose that grades serve is administrative, and there are many uses of grades for this purpose. These include: admission of students to nursing programs, at the entry level and for admission to higher degree programs; progression of students in a program, for continuation in the nursing program and decisions about completion of sequential nursing courses; graduation; probation of students; eligibility of students to complete specialized programs, such as nurse practitioner certification programs; awarding scholarships and fellowships; awarding honors and determining acceptance into honor societies, such as Sigma Theta Tau International; as a part of program evaluation studies; and reporting to employers.

The third broad purpose of using grades is for guidance and counseling decisions. Grades may be used to make decisions about courses to select, including more advanced courses to take, remedial courses that might be helpful, and what courses to take next; decide on types of assistance needed by students, for example, reading, study, and test-taking skills; counsel students; and assist students in making career choices, including a change in direction of one's career. These purposes of grades are summarized in Table 13.1.

CRITICISMS OF GRADES

Although grades serve many purposes, there are just as many criticisms of them as there are uses. Nitko (1996) identified a number of these criticisms that are applicable to grading in nursing programs. Responses are offered to each criticism.

Table 13.1 Purposes of Grades

Instructional
    Achievement of students in learning activities, clinical practice, and
        nursing courses
    Progress reports to students

Administrative
    Admission
    Progression
    Graduation
    Probation
    Eligibility to complete specialized courses
    Scholarships and fellowships
    Honors and eligibility for honor societies
    Program evaluation
    Reporting to employers

Guidance and counseling
    Courses to take—advanced, remedial, and sequential
    Assistance needed by students
    Career decisions

1. *Grades are meaningless because of the diversity across schools of nursing, course faculty, clinical teachers, and preceptors.* This criticism suggests a need to improve grading practices in nursing programs, use a consistent grading system across sections of nursing courses and for grading clinical practice, orient more carefully course faculty to grading, develop a comprehensive system for orienting part-time clinical faculty and preceptors involved in clinical teaching of nursing students in how to evaluate learning and determine grades, and engage teachers in discussions about evaluation and grading practices and values and attitudes about grading.

2. *A single symbol, such as an A or a pass, does not adequately represent the complex details associated with achievement in nursing courses.* Grades, however, are not intended to fulfill this need; it is acknowledged that grades do not reflect every detail of the student's learning in a course, nor every accomplishment. Grades are a summarization of achievements over a period of time.

3. *Grades are not important.* Although a grade is only a symbol of achievement, Nitko (1996) emphasized that grades are important. The multiple ways that grades are used to arrive at educational decisions suggest that they are important to students, nursing programs, and others. In

addition, grades and overall grade point average may predict later achievement, such as performance on the NCLEX. Although some have argued that the most valuable outcomes are intangible, grades, nevertheless, remain important indicators of overall achievement.

4. *Grades are less important than self-evaluations.* Nitko (1996) argued that both self-evaluation and grades are essential, not one or the other. Grades by the teacher "help individuals to realistically evaluate themselves" (p. 327).

5. *Grades are unnecessary.* In most educational settings, grades can not be eliminated. They are necessary to serve the purposes set forth earlier.

6. *Grades are ineffective motivators.* For some students, grades are effective motivators; for others, this may not be true. A certain level of performance, however, is essential for progression in nursing programs and later educational decisions. Some students are more motivated by grades than others.

7. *Low grades discourage students.* While lower grades may be discouraging and stressful for students, they are essential for determining progression in a nursing program. Nursing programs are accountable to the profession and to society for graduating students who have the knowledge and skills for managing the health needs of clients. Not all entering students have the ability to acquire this knowledge and these skills. Low grades are important for counseling students and suggesting remedial instruction; failing grades indicate when students have not met the criteria for continuing in the nursing program.

Ebel and Frisbie (1991) recommended that instead of criticizing grades, teachers should assign them more carefully, devote more attention to improving their validity, and develop better mechanisms for interpreting grades to others.

TYPES OF GRADING SYSTEMS

There are different types of grading systems or methods of reporting grades. Most teachers use a letter system for grading, A, B, C, D, E or A, B, C, D, F, which may be combined with "+" and "−." The integers 5, 4, 3, 2, and 1 (or 9 through 1) also may be used. These two systems of grading are convenient to use, yield grades that are able to be averaged within a course and across courses, and present the grade concisely. Grading standards and the meaning of the letter or number, however, may vary with the teacher, nursing course, clinical practice component, and school of nursing. There may be a lack of clear guidelines for determining the grade and lack of a common understanding of the achievement represented by each grade. A grade of "A" in one nursing course may reflect different standards than this same grade in another nursing course.

Grades also may be indicated by percentages (100, 99, 98, . . .). Most schools use percentages as a basis for assigning letter grades (Bott, 1996). For example, 90% to 100% may represent an A, 80 to 89% a B, and so forth. In some nursing programs, these percentages for each letter grade are higher, for instance, 92% to 100% for an A, 83% to 91% a B, 75% to 82% a C, 66% to 74% a D, and 65% and below an E or F. In most cases, test scores should not be converted to grades for the purpose of later computing a final average grade. Instead, the teacher should record actual test scores and then combine them into a composite score that can be converted to a final grade.

Another type of grading system is two-dimensional; these are categories, pass–fail, satisfactory–unsatisfactory, and credit–no credit. For determining clinical grades, some nursing programs add a third honors category resulting in three levels: honors–pass–fail. One advantage of a two-dimensional grading system is that the grade is not calculated in the grade point average. This allows students to take new courses and explore different areas of learning without concern about the grades in these courses affecting the overall grade point average. This also may be viewed as a disadvantage, however, in that clinical performance in a nursing course graded on a pass–fail basis is not calculated as part of the overall course grade. A pass indicates that students met the clinical objectives or demonstrated satisfactory performance of the clinical competencies. Gronlund and Linn (1990) emphasized that a pass-fail system is valuable for courses in which students are expected to attain mastery. When students need to master the objectives and acquire certain knowledge and skills before receiving credit for the course, then a "simple pass is all that is needed to indicate mastery" (p. 431). This rationale is consistent with clinical courses based on the pass-fail system. These different systems for grading clinical practice are discussed in a later section of the chapter.

Grade Point Average

One other dimension of a grading system involves converting the letter grade to a grade point system for calculating the grade point average (GPA) or quality point average (QPA). Some schools use a 4-point system; others include plus and minus grades. Grades in a 4-point system are typically:

A = 4 points per credit (or unit)
B = 3 points per credit
C = 2 points per credit
D = 1 point per credit
F = 0 points per credit

If a student took two 3-credit courses and one 6-credit nursing course and received an A in one of the 3-credit courses, a C in the other, and a B in the 6-credit course, the grade point average would be:

A = 4 points/credit = 4 points × 3 credits = 12 points
C = 2 points/credit = 2 points × 3 credits = 6 points
B = 3 points/credit = 3 points × 6 credits = 18 points

36 ÷ 12 (credits) = 3.0.

The letter system for grading also may include plus and minus grades as presented in Table 13.2.

ASSIGNING LETTER GRADES

Because most schools of nursing use the letter system for grading nursing courses, this framework will be used for discussing how to assign grades. These principles, however, are applicable to the other grading systems as well. There are two major considerations in assigning letter grades: deciding what to include in the grade and selecting a grading framework.

Deciding What to Include in the Grade

As a first principle, grades for nursing courses should reflect student achievement in them; they should not be biased by the teacher's own values, beliefs, and attitudes. If the student did not attend class or appeared to be inattentive during lectures, this behavior should not be incorporated in the course grade unless criteria were established at the outset for class attendance and participation. In determining the grade for a course, including clinical practice, the grade should indicate students' achievement of course objectives and how well they performed in the clinical setting based on the objectives or competencies set for clinical practice. "If letter grades are to serve as valid indicators of achievement, they must be based on valid measures of achievement" (Gronlund & Linn, 1990, p. 437).

This process of developing valid measures of achievement begins at

Table 13.2 Plus-and-Minus System

Grade	Description	Grade Points
A	Outstanding	4.0
A-		3.7
B+		3.3
B	Very good	3.0
B-		2.7
C+		2.3
C	Average	2.0
C-		1.7
D+		1.3
D	Minimally passing	1.0
D-		0.7
F	Failure	0.0

From P. A. Bott, (1996). *Testing and Assessment in Occupational and Technical Education* (p.194). Boston: Allyn and Bacon. Copyright 1996 by Allyn and Bacon. Adapted with permission.

the point of establishing the objectives for the course and for clinical practice and developing tests and evaluation methods to measure the attainment of these objectives. These tests and evaluation methods, then, form the basis for determining the student's grade. The weight given to each test and evaluation strategy in the grade is specified by the teacher according to the emphasis of the objectives and content measured by them. Tests and other evaluation methods measuring important objectives and content, for which more time was probably spent in the instruction, should receive greater weight in the course grade. For example, midterm examination in a community health nursing course should be given more weight in the course grade than a paper students completed about community resources for a family under their care.

Selecting a Grading Framework

To give meaning to the grades assigned, the teacher needs a grading framework or frame of reference. There are three grading frameworks used to assign meaning to grades: criterion-referenced, also referred to as grading with absolute standards; norm-referenced, or grading with relative standards; and self-referenced, grading based on the growth of the student (Nitko, 1996). Criterion- and norm-referenced evaluation methods were described in earlier chapters; these same concepts apply to grading frameworks. Grades are symbols that indicate a judgment about the student's achievement in relation to (a) predefined objectives or knowledge and skills mastered, without regard to the achievement of other students; (b) how well other students in the class or clinical practice performed; and (c) the student's own development of knowledge and skills in the course.

The decision as to which of these frameworks to use is the teacher's, although there should be consistency across different sections of a nursing course and for clinical courses; it is difficult to mandate the use of one framework for all courses in the nursing program because of differences in teaching and evaluation philosophies among teachers and varying instructional approaches used in courses. Consistency in grading clinical practice, however, is essential, for grades might vary considerably if assigned based on achievement of the clinical objectives alone; if each student's performance is compared to others in the clinical group; or if the progress of the student in developing clinical competencies is the sole basis for assigning the grade.

Criterion-Referenced Grading

In criterion-referenced grading, grades are based on the student's achievement of predetermined objectives, mastery of content, or performance of a defined set of competencies. Students who achieve more of the objectives, acquire more knowledge, and can perform more competencies or with greater proficiency receive higher grades. The meaning assigned to grades, then, is based on these absolute standards, without regard to the achievement of other students. Using this frame of reference for grading means it is possible for all students to achieve an A or B in a course, if they meet these standards, or a D or F if they do not meet them. Table 13.3 illustrates criterion-referenced grading.

FIXED-PERCENT METHOD

There are several ways of assigning grades using a criterion-referenced system. One way is called the fixed-percent method. Each component of the grade is given a percent-correct, or percentage of the total points possible (Nitko, 1996, p. 341). For instance, the student might have achieved a score of 21 out of 25 on a quiz, or 84%. The percentages are then converted to a letter grade at the end of the course. With all grading systems students need to be informed how the grade will be assigned. If the fixed-percent method is used, the scale for converting percentages to letter

Table 13.3 Grading Frameworks

Grade	Criterion referenced	Norm referenced	Self-referenced
A	All objectives met High level of performance of all competencies	Achievement/ performance far exceeds average of group (e.g., other students in class)	Made significant progress Gained significant amount of knowledge and skills Performed significantly higher than expected
B	All essential objectives met and at least half of the other objectives High level of performance of most competencies	Above the average of the group	Made progress and gained knowledge and skills Performed higher than expected
C	All essential objectives met Ability to perform most competencies reflecting criteria	Average in comparison with the group	Made progress in most areas Met performance level expected by teacher
D	One half or more of essential objectives met Unable to perform some essential competencies	Below the average of the group	Made some gains Did not meet level of performance for which capable
F	Most essential objectives not achieved Most competencies not able to be performed	Failing achievement/ performance in comparison with the group	Made no gains Performance significantly below capability

Note: This table is an adaptation of selected ideas from A. J. Nitko (1996). *Educational Assessment of Students* (2nd ed.). Upper Saddle River, NJ: Prentice Hall. Copyright 1996 by Prentice Hall. Adapted with permission.

grades should be communicated to students and adhered to in the grading process.

The fixed-percent method may be used to combine scores from the various components of the grade, for example, tests, quizzes, papers, and other evaluation methods, into a single composite score. The first step, and an important one, is to assign weights to each of the components of the grade. How much weight should be given in the grade to each test and other type of evaluation method used in the course? An example follows:

Paper on nursing interventions	10%
Papers critiquing issues in clinical practice	20%
Quizzes	10%
Midterm examination	20%
Portfolio	20%
Final examination	20%
	100%

In determining the composite score for the course, the student's percentage for each of these components is multiplied by the weight and summed; the sum is then divided by the sum of the weights. This procedure is illustrated in Table 13.4.

One major limitation with the fixed-percent method is that some of the tests and evaluation methods used in a course may be more difficult than others, and the teacher may not know this in advance to weigh them accordingly (Nitko,1996); this is particularly true of new assignments in a course. They also may be much easier and require less time and effort than planned originally when the grading scheme was decided upon. With this method, the percentage that the assignment counts toward the grade may not reflect its difficulty or ease of completion. This is often a concern for students who complain that a difficult assignment requiring extensive time counted less in the course grade than other evaluation methods.

TOTAL-POINTS METHOD

The second method of assigning grades in a criterion-referenced system is the total-points method. Each component of the grade is assigned specific points, for instance, a paper may be assigned 100 points and the midterm examination 200 points. The number of points assigned reflects the weights given the components within the course, what each one is "worth." An example follows:

Table 13.4 Fixed-Percent Method for Grading Nursing Courses

Components of course grade and weights	%
Paper on nursing interventions	10
Papers critiquing issues in clinical practice	20
Quizzes	10
Midterm examination	20
Portfolio	20
Final examination	20

Student	Intervention paper (wt. = 10%)	Issue papers (wt. = 20%)	Quizzes (wt. = 10%)	Midterm (wt. = 20%)	Portfolio (wt. = 20%)	Final (wt.= 20%)
Mary	85	94	98	92	94	91
Jane	76	76	63	79	70	79
Bob	82	86	89	81	80	83

Composite score for Mary:
[10(85) + 20(94) + 10(98) + 20(92) + 20(94) + 20(91)] ÷ 100 (sum of weights) = 92.5%

Composite score for Jane:
[10(76) + 20(78) + 10(63) + 20(79) + 20(79) + 20(70)] ÷ 100 = 75.1%

Composite score for Bob:
[10(82) + 20(86) + 10(89) + 20(81) + 20(80) + 20(83)] ÷ 100 = 83.1%

Paper on nursing interventions	100 points
Papers critiquing issues in clinical practice	200 points
Quizzes	100 points
Midterm examination	200 points
Portfolio	200 points
Final examination	200 points
	1,000 points

The points for each component are not converted to a letter grade; instead, the grades are assigned according to the number of total points accumulated at the end of the course. At that time, letter grades are assigned based on the points needed for each grade. For example,

Grade	Points
A	900–1,000
B	800–899
C	700–799
D	600–699
F	0–599

Norm-Referenced Grading

In a norm-referenced grading system, using relative standards, grades are assigned by comparing a student's performance with others in the class. Students who perform better than their peers receive higher grades (Nitko, 1996). In using a norm-referenced system, the teacher decides on the reference group against which to compare student performance. Should students be compared to others in the course? To students in their section only of the course? Or, to students who completed the course the prior semester or previous year? One issue with norm-referenced grading is that high performance in a particular group may not be indicative of mastery of the content nor what students have learned; it reflects instead a student's standing in a group. Table 13.3 illustrates norm-referenced grading.

Three methods of assigning grades using a norm-referenced system are grading (a) on the curve, (b) based on the distribution gap, or (c) by using standard deviations. Grading on the curve refers to the score distribution curve. In this method, students' scores are rank-ordered from highest to lowest, and grades are assigned according to the rank order. One issue with this method is that the teacher needs to decide on the quotas for each grading category, an arbitrary decision (Ebel & Frisbie, 1991). What proportion of the grades should be As? Bs? and so forth. For example,

Grade	Percentage
A	Top 15% of students
B	Next 30%
C	Next 30%
D	Next 15%
F	Lowest 10%

After the quotas are set, grades are assigned without considering actual achievement; for instance, the top 15% of the students may receive an A, but their scores may be close to the next 30% who received a B. The students assigned a D and an F may in fact have acquired sufficient knowledge in the course, but had lower scores in comparison with the other students.

With the distribution-gap method, students are ranked in order of the frequency distribution of the scores. Gaps, a series of scores not obtained by any of the students, are identified in the frequency distribution; grades are then assigned. Scores above the top gap, for instance, are assigned As, and above the second gap Bs, continuing until all the grade ranges are determined. This method shares many of the drawbacks of grading on the curve.

The third method is based on standard deviations. With this method, the teacher determines the cut-off points with equal intervals for each grade. The following steps for using the standard deviation method were specified by Ebel and Frisbie (1991):

1. Do a frequency distribution for the composite scores.
2. Compute the median and standard deviation.
3. Determine cut-off points for the C grade range by adding $1/2$ of the standard deviation to the median and subtracting $1/2$ of the standard deviation from the median.
4. Add one standard deviation to the upper cut-off number of the C range to find the A and B cut-off scores.
5. Subtract the same amount from the lower cut-off number of the C range to identify the D and F cut-off scores.
6. Review borderline cases; consider the quality of individual assignments and other evaluation data to "decide if borderline cases should be raised or lowered." (p. 280)

Self-Referenced Grading

Self-referenced grading is based on standards of growth and change in the student. With this method, grades are assigned by comparing the student's performance with the teacher's perceptions of the student's capabilities (Nitko, 1996, p. 336). Did the student achieve at a higher level than deemed capable, regardless of the knowledge and competencies acquired? Did the student improve performance throughout the course?

Table 13.3 compares self-referencing with criterion- and norm-referenced grading. One major problem with this method is the unreliability of the teacher's perceptions of student capability and growth. A second issue occurs with students who enter the course or clinical practice with a high level of achievement and proficiency in many of the clinical competencies. These students may have the least amount of growth and change, but nevertheless exit the course with the highest achievement and clinical competency.

GRADING CLINICAL PRACTICE

Arriving at grades for clinical practice is difficult because of the nature of clinical practice and need for judgments about performance. The many issues facing faculty in evaluating clinical practice and rating performance were described in chapters 10 and 11. Many teachers constantly revise their clinical evaluation instruments and seek new ways of grading clinical practice; while these changes may create a fairer grading system, they will not eliminate the problems inherent in judging performance in the clinical setting.

The different types of grading systems described earlier may be used for grading clinical practice. In general, these include multidimensional systems such as letter grades, A through F; integers, 5 through 1; and percentages. Grading systems for clinical practice also may be two-dimensional, including the categories pass–fail, satisfactory–unsatisfactory, and met–did not meet the clinical objectives. Some programs add a third category, honors, to acknowledge performance that exceeds the level required. With any of these grading systems, it is not always easy to summarize the multiple types of evaluation data collected about the student's performance into a symbol representing a grade. This is true even in a pass–fail system; it may be difficult to arrive at a judgment as to pass or fail based on the evaluation data and the circumstances associated with the student's clinical practice.

Regardless of the grading system for clinical practice, there are two criteria to be met: (a) the evaluation methods for collecting data about student performance should reflect the clinical objectives and competencies for which a grade will be assigned, and (b) students must be aware of and understand how their clinical practice will be evaluated and graded.

Decisions about assigning letter grades for clinical practice are the same as those that arise in grading any course: deciding what to include in the clinical grade and selecting a grading framework. The first consideration relates to the evaluation methods used in the course to provide data for determining the clinical grade. Some of these evaluation strategies are designated by the teacher as summative evaluation methods, thereby providing a source of information for including in the clinical grade. Other strategies, though, are used in clinical practice for feedback only, and not incorporated in the grade.

The second consideration is the grading framework. Will achievement in clinical practice be graded from A to F? 5 to 1? Pass–fail? Or variations of these? The second related question is: How will the clinical grade be included in the course grade, if at all?

Pass–Fail

Categories for grading clinical practice, such as pass–fail and satisfactory–unsatisfactory, have some advantages over a multidimensional system, although there are disadvantages as well. Pass–fail, for instance, places greater emphasis on giving feedback to the learner because only two categories of performance need to be determined. Faculty using this grading system may be more inclined to provide continual feedback to learners because they do not have to ultimately differentiate performance according to four or five levels of proficiency, such as with a letter system for grading clinical practice. High-quality performance exceeding the requirements and expectations, though, is not reflected in the grade for clinical practice unless a third category is included: honors–pass–fail.

A pass-fail system requires only two types of judgment about clinical performance. Do the evaluation data indicate that the student has met the objective, demonstrating satisfactory performance of that competency to indicate a pass? Or, do the data suggest that the performance is not at a satisfactory level to pass the competency? Arriving at a judgment as to pass or fail is often easier for the teacher than using the same evaluation information for deciding on five levels of performance. A letter system for grading clinical practice, though, acknowledges the different levels of clinical proficiency students may have demonstrated in their clinical practice.

Early on in the use of the pass–fail system teachers expressed concern about the effect of pass–fail grading on applications to nursing programs as students continued their education. Most programs, however, consider overall grade point average for admission, regardless of whether the clinical grade is incorporated in it or assigned by the pass–fail method.

One disadvantage of pass–fail for grading clinical practice is inability to include a clinical grade into the course grade. One strategy is to separate nursing courses into two components for grading, one for the classroom and related experiences and the second for clinical practice, designated as pass–fail, even though the course is considered as a whole. Typically, guidelines for the course indicate that students must pass the clinical component to pass the course. A second mechanism is to offer two separate courses with the clinical course graded on a pass–fail basis. Karns and Nowotny (1991) reported, from their survey of BSN programs, that a pass–fail grading system was used in 61% of the clinical courses that were separate courses, and in 59% that combined theory and clinical practice into one course grade (pp. 208–209). They also reported that 91% of the faculty using a pass–fail system for grading clinical practice were satisfied with it, compared with 56% of those grading clinical practice based on a letter system.

Once the grading system is determined, there are varied ways of using it to arrive at the clinical grade. In one method, the grade is assigned based on the clinical objectives or competencies attained by the student. To use this method, the teacher may want to designate some of the objectives or competencies as critical for achievement. Table 13.3 provides guidelines for converting the clinical objectives or competencies into letter grades within a criterion-referenced system. For example, an A might be assigned if all of the clinical objectives were met; a B might be assigned if all of the objectives designated by faculty as critical behaviors and at least half of the other objectives were met.

For pass–fail grading, faculty may indicate that all objectives or competencies must be met to pass the course, or may designate critical objectives or competencies required for passing the course. In both methods, the clinical evaluation strategies provide the data for determining if the student's performance reflects achievement of the competencies. These evaluation strategies may or may not be graded separately as part of the course grade.

Another way of arriving at the clinical grade is to base it on the designated evaluation strategies. In this system the clinical evaluation methods become the source of data for the grade. For example,

Paper on analysis of clinical practice issue	10%
Process recording	5%
Conference presentation	10%
Case analysis (paper and presentation)	10%
Portfolio	25%
Rating scale (of performance)	40%

In this illustration, the clinical grade is computed according to the evaluation methods. Observation of performance, and the rating on the clinical evaluation instrument, is only a portion of the clinical grade. One advantage of this approach is that it incorporates into the grade the summative evaluation strategies competed by students.

If pass-fail is used for grading clinical practice, the grade might be computed as follows:

Paper on analysis of clinical practice issue	10%
Process recording	5%
Conference presentation	10%
Case analysis (paper and presentation)	10%
Portfolio	25%
Clinical examination	40%
Rating scale (of performance)	Pass required

This discussion of grading clinical practice suggests a variety of mechanisms that are appropriate. The teacher must make it clear to students and others how evaluation and grading will be carried out in clinical practice.

Failing Clinical Practice

Teachers will be faced with determining when students have not met the clinical objectives, have not performed satisfactorily in the clinical setting to demonstrate competency, and therefore fail the clinical course or clinical component of a nursing course. There are some principles to be adhered to in developing and implementing a system for evaluating and grading clinical practice that will be of value if a student fails a clinical course or has the potential for failing it.

1. The evaluation methods used in a clinical course, how each will be graded if at all, and how the clinical grade will be assigned should be in writing and communicated to students. The practices of the teacher in evaluating and grading clinical performance should reflect this written information.

2. If failing clinical practice, whether in a pass–fail or letter system, means failing the nursing course, this should be stated as such and communicated to students in writing. In a letter grade system, the policy should include the letter-grade representing a failure in clinical practice, for instance, less than a C grade.

3. Problems in clinical performance, in relation to achieving the clinical objectives or competencies, when identified by the teacher should be discussed early on with the student. The observations made by the teacher and other evaluation data should be shared with the student who should participate in these discussions. The discussions should not take the form of the teacher "telling the student." There should be documentation of the evaluation data and the discussions held with the student. Remedial instruction should be planned and documented to enable the student to develop competencies further and correct deficiencies.

4. Students should sign any written clinical evaluation documents indicating that they have read the comments; their signatures do not mean they agree with them. Students should, however, have an opportunity to write in their own comments. These documents are valuable at the end of the semester for students who have failed the clinical course (Brooke, 1994, p. 253).

5. If the remedial instruction is ineffective, however, in moving the student toward achieving the clinical objectives or competencies, Graveley and Stanley (1993) recommend writing a plan that includes: (a) the clinical deficiencies (lack of knowledge for practice, deficiencies in performing skills, areas of practice in which the student is unsafe, and so forth) and "strategies to bring the student to the required level of performance;" (b) a statement that one "good or poor" performance will not constitute a

passing or failing clinical grade and sustained improvement is needed; and (c) a statement that the remedial instruction and strategies included in the plan do not supplant satisfactory performance by the student of the clinical objectives by the end of the course (p. 136).

6. Students with the potential of failing clinical practice may have other problems affecting their performance; teachers should refer students to counseling and other support services, and not attempt to provide these resources themselves. Attempting to counsel the student and help the student cope with other problems may bias the teacher and influence judgment of clinical performance.

7. As the clinical course progresses, the teacher should give feedback to the student documenting specifically the observations made, other evaluation data collected, and additional teaching strategies used. The content of these discussions should be recorded.

8. There should be a policy in the nursing program about actions to be taken if the student is unsafe in clinical practice. If the practice is safe, however, but does not meet the clinical objectives, the student "must be allowed to continue in the course" (Graveley & Stanley, 1993, p. 137). This is the case because the clinical objectives are specified for achievement at the *end* of the course, not during it.

9. There should be a policy in the nursing program for student-initiated academic review. Students should be aware of the policy and mechanism for initiating it if they fail the clinical course. Graveley and Stanley (1993) indicated that if the student does not initiate the academic review process, the school of nursing is not at fault (p. 135).

10. In cases involving failure in clinical practice, the "critical issue is ensuring due process" for the student (Graveley & Stanley, 1993, p. 135). The discussions held with students in jeopardy of failing clinical practice should focus on the student's inability to meet the clinical objectives and perform the specified competencies, and not on the teacher's perceptions of the student's intelligence and overall ability. In addition, these opinions about the student's ability in general should not be discussed with anyone.

11. Other legal requirements to be met when supervising a nursing student with the potential of failing clinical practice include the following: (a) The policies and established procedures for student dismissal from clinical practice and academic failures in clinical courses must be adhered to; (b) the student must be notified that she or he has failed the clinical course and of the consequences of this failure, such as dismissal from the nursing program or repeating the clinical course; and (c) the student should be informed of the reasons for the failure/dismissal and "encouraged to follow any other academic review procedures contained in the catalog" (Graveley & Stanley, 1993, p. 136).

GRADING SOFTWARE

A number of the procedures for determining grades are time-consuming especially for a large class of students. Although a calculator may be used, a spreadsheet program for a personal computer makes it easier to record and calculate the grades. There also are a number of grading software programs on the market that include a premade spreadsheet for grading purposes, have different grading frameworks that may be used for calculating the grade, and enable the teacher to carry out the tasks needed for grading. With this software, the teacher can print out grading reports for the class as a whole and individual students. Some even calculate test statistics. Not all grading software programs are of high quality, and all should be reviewed prior to purchase.

SUMMARY

This chapter introduced concepts of grading or marking. Grading is defined as the use of symbols, for instance, the letters A through F, to report student achievement. Grading is for summative purposes, indicating through the use of symbols how well the student met the course and clinical objectives. Grades need to be based on careful evaluation practices, valid and reliable test results, and multiple evaluation measures. No grade should be determined on one evaluation method or one assignment completed by students; grades reflect instead a combination of various tests and other evaluation methods.

There are different types of grading systems or methods of reporting grades: the letters A, B, C, D, E or A, B, C, D, F, which may be combined with "+" and "−"; integers 5, 4, 3, 2, and 1 (or 9 through 1); percentages; and categories such as pass–fail and satisfactory–unsatisfactory. Advantages and disadvantages of pass-fail for grading clinical practice were discussed in the chapter.

Two major considerations in assigning letter grades are deciding what to include in the grade and selecting a grading framework. The weight given to each test and evaluation strategy in the grade is specified by the teacher according to the emphasis of the objectives and content measured by the test. To give meaning to the grades assigned, the teacher needs a grading framework: criterion-referenced, also referred to as grading with absolute standards; norm-referenced, or grading with relative standards; or self-referenced, grading based on the growth of the student.

One final concept described in the chapter was grading clinical practice and guidelines for working with students with the potential for failing the clinical course. These guidelines give direction to teachers in establishing sound grading policies and procedures and following them when working with students in clinical practice.

REFERENCES

Bott, P. A. (1996). *Testing and assessment in occupational and technical education*. Boston: Allyn and Bacon

Brooke, P. S. (1994). Comment on Orchard's "clinical evaluation procedures." *Journal of Nursing Education, 33*, 252–253.

Ebel, R. L., & Frisbie, D. A. (1991). *Essential of educational measurement* (5th ed.). Englewood Cliffs, NJ: Prentice Hall.

Graveley, E. A., & Stanley, M. (1993). A clinical failure: What the courts tell us. *Journal of Nursing Education, 32*, 135–137.

Gronlund, N. E., & Linn, R. L. (1990). *Measurement and evaluation in teaching* (6th ed.). New York: Macmillan.

Karns, P., & Nowotny, M. (1991). Clinical structure and evaluation in baccalaureate schools of nursing. *Journal of Nursing Education, 30*, 207–211.

Nitko, A. J. (1996). *Educational assessment of students* (2nd ed.). Englewood Cliffs, NJ: Prentice Hall.

14

Social, Ethical, and Legal Issues

Educational testing and evaluation are growing in use and importance for society in general and nursing in particular. One only has to read the comic strips and cartoons published in newspapers and popular magazines to appreciate the prevalence of testing and evaluation in contemporary American society. From the moment of birth, when we are weighed, measured, and rated according to the Apgar scale, throughout all of our educational and work experiences, and even in our personal and social lives, we are used to being tested and evaluated. In addition, nursing and other professional disciplines have come under increasing public pressure to be accountable for the quality of educational programs and the competency of its practitioners, and testing and evaluation often are used to provide evidence of quality and competence. Sometimes the public demand for this information results in the preparation of poor tests or the unwise use of existing tests (Ebel & Frisbie, 1991).

With increasing use of evaluation and testing comes intensified interest and concern about fairness, appropriateness, and impact. This chapter discusses selected social, ethical, and legal issues related to testing and evaluation practices in nursing education.

SOCIAL ISSUES

Testing has tremendous social impact because test scores can have positive and negative consequences for individuals. Tests can provide information to assist in decision making; some of those decisions have more importance to society and to individuals than other decisions. The licensure of drivers is a good example. Written and performance tests provide information for making decisions about who may drive a vehicle. Society has a vested interest in the outcome because a bad decision can affect the safety of a great many people. Licensure to drive a vehicle also may be an important issue to an individual; some jobs require the employee to drive a car or truck, and a person who lacks a valid operator's license will not have access to these employment opportunities.

Tests also are used to sort individuals into occupational roles. This sorting has important implications because a person's occupation to some extent determines status and economic and political power. Because modern societies heavily depend upon scientific knowledge and technical competence, occupational role selection to a significant degree is based on what individuals know and can do. Educational institutions, therefore, have an important social function of matching persons and occupational roles through control of academic credentials (Berlak et al., 1992).

The way in which schools should select candidates for occupational roles, however, is a matter of controversy. Some individuals and cultural groups hold the view that schools should provide equality of opportunity and access to educational programs. Others believe that equal opportunity is not sufficient to allow some categories of people to overcome discrimination and oppression that has handicapped ability and opportunity. Those who hold this view believe that affirmative action and public policy changes are required to guarantee equality of outcome (Berlak et al., 1992).

Decisions about which individuals should be admitted to a school of nursing are important because of nursing's commitment to the good of society and to the health and welfare of present and future patients (American Nurses Association, 1995). Teachers must select individuals for admission to nursing programs who are likely to practice nursing competently and safely; tests frequently are used to assist teachers to select candidates for admission. Improper use of testing, or misinterpretation of test scores, can result in two types of poor admission decisions. If an individual is selected who is later found to be incompetent to practice nursing safely, the public may suffer harm; if an individual who would be competent to practice nursing is not admitted, that individual is denied access to an occupational role. The use of testing in employment situations and for the purpose of professional certification can produce similar results. The consequences for the test-takers are great because the decisions made will affect economic opportunities and career paths (Ebel & Frisbie, 1991); employers have a stake in the decisions made because they are responsible for ensuring the competence of their employees (Dowd, 1995). Selection decisions therefore have social implications for individuals as well as for society as a whole.

Although educational and occupational uses of testing are growing in use and importance, the public often expresses concerns about testing. Some of these concerns are rational and relevant; others are unjustified.

Test Bias

One common concern is that tests are biased or unfair to some groups of test-takers. A major purpose of testing is to discriminate among people, that is, to identify important differences among them with regard to their knowledge, skills, or attitudes. To the extent that differences in scores represent real differences in achievement of objectives, this discrimination is not necessarily unfair (Nitko, 1996). In most cases unfairness results from the improper use of test results, not the test itself (Ebel & Frisbie, 1991). For example, if a test is found to discriminate between men and women on variables that are not relevant to educational or occupational success, the use of that test to select applicants for admission or employment would be unfair (Lyman, 1991; Nitko, 1996). Thus, the question of test bias is really one of test validity, the degree to which the test is relevant for the purpose for which it is used.

Test bias also has been defined as the differential validity of a test score for a definable subgroup of test-takers, so that a given score does not have the same meaning for all students who took that test (Hambleton, 1989). The teacher may interpret a low test score to mean inadequate knowledge of the content, but there may be a relevant subgroup of individuals, for example, students with learning disabilities, for whom that score interpretation is not accurate. A learning-disabled student may have earned a low score because of insufficient time to complete the test, not because of incomplete or incorrect knowledge (Klisch, 1994).

Individual test items also can discriminate against subgroups of test-takers, such as students from ethnic minority groups. Test items are considered to be biased when students of different subgroups but equal ability, as evidenced by equal total test scores, perform differently on the item. Item bias exists in two forms, cultural bias and structural bias.

A culturally biased item contains references to a particular culture and is more likely to be answered incorrectly by students from a minority group. An example of a culturally biased test item follows:

While discussing her health patterns with the nurse, Ms. A says that she enjoys all of the following leisure activities. Which one is an aerobic activity?

    a. Attending ballet performances
    b. Cultivating house plants
    c. Line dancing
    d. Singing in the church choir

The correct answer is "line dancing," but students for whom English is a second language (ESL) and other minority students may be unfamiliar with this term and therefore may not select this response. In this case, an incorrect response may mean that the student is unfamiliar with this type of dancing, not that the student is unable to differentiate between aerobic and anaerobic activities. Careful peer review of test items for discernible bias, as discussed in chapter 8, allows the teacher to reword items to remove references to U. S. or English literature, music, art, history, customs, or regional terminology that are not essential to the nursing content being tested. The inclusion of jokes, puns, and other forms of humor also may contribute to cultural bias, as these forms of expression may not be interpreted correctly by ESL students. It is appropriate, however, to include cultural references that are essential to safe nursing practice. Students and graduate nurses must be culturally competent if they are to meet the needs of patients from a variety of cultures. For example, in order to communicate effectively with patients and families, nurses must know the meaning of eye contact in different cultures (Klisch, 1994).

A test item with structural bias is poorly written. It may be lengthy, unclear, or awkwardly worded. Structurally biased items can bewilder all students, but they are more likely to discriminate against ESL students or those with learning disabilities, who can be confused more easily by wording or grammar (Klisch, 1994). Additionally, students from minority cultures may be less likely than dominant-culture students to ask the test proctor to clarify a poorly written item; it is inappropriate to question a teacher in some cultures. Following the general rules for writing test items in chapter 3 will help the teacher to avoid structural bias.

An evaluation practice that helps to protect students from potential bias is anonymous or blinded scoring and grading. The process is similar to that of peer review of manuscripts and grant proposals: the teacher is unaware of the student's identity until the end of the course. Students choose a code number or name at the beginning of a course and record that code on every test and written assignment; the teacher does not know the identity of the student whose test or paper is being scored. Scores are recorded according to codes, and it is only at the end of the course that students' names and codes are revealed. This method of grading and scoring has been suggested as a way to avoid the halo effects of the teacher's preconceived assessments of students based on their previous experience or class behavior (McDaniel, 1994).

Grade and Test Score Inflation

Another common criticism of testing concerns the general trend toward inflation of test scores and grades at all educational levels. Grade inflation distorts the meaning of test scores, making it difficult for teachers to use them wisely in decision making. If an A is intended to represent exceptional or superior performance, then all students cannot earn As, because if everyone is exceptional then no one is. Where there is no distribution of scores or grades, there is little value in testing. Lyman (1991) called this trend the "Lake Wobegon effect," referring to the fictional town created by humorist Garrison Keillor in which "all the children are above average" (p. 43). If everyone was above average, however, it would be virtually impossible to select the winner of an academic scholarship or to reward superior job performance with a merit raise.

One factor contributing to grade inflation may be the increasing pressure of accountability for educational outcomes. When the effectiveness of a teacher's instruction is judged on the basis of students' test performance and when there are significant negative consequences of low scores, there is strong temptation to "teach to the test" (Ebel & Frisbie, 1991; Lyman, 1991). Teaching to the test may involve using actual test items as practice exercises, distributing copies of a previously used test for review and then using the same test, or focusing exclusively on test content in teaching. It is important, however, to distinguish between teaching to the test and purposeful teaching of content to be sampled by the test and practice of relevant test-taking skills. Nursing faculty members who understand the NCLEX test plan and ensure that their nursing curricula include content and learning activities that will enable students to be successful on the NCLEX are not teaching to the test.

Effect of Tests and Grades on Self-Esteem

Some critics of tests claim that testing results in emotional or psychological harm to students. The concern is that tests threaten students and make them anxious, fearful, and discouraged, resulting in harm to students' self-esteem. There is no empirical evidence to support these claims. Feelings of anxiety about an upcoming test are normal and helpful to the extent that they motivate students to prepare thoroughly in order to demonstrate their best performance. Since testing is a common life event, learning how to cope with these challenges is a necessary part of student development. In some cases, test anxiety is elevated to harmful levels; this problem cannot be solved, however, by eliminating tests (Ebel & Frisbie, 1991).

Although it is probably true that a certain level of self-esteem is necessary before a student will attempt the challenges associated with nursing education, the authors do not believe that students must have high self-esteem before they can be expected to perform well. In fact, if students are able to perform at their best, their self-esteem is enhanced. An important part of a teacher's role is to prepare students to do well on tests by helping them improve their study and test-taking skills and learn to manage their anxiety.

Testing As a Means of Social Control

All societies sanction some form of social control of behavior; some teachers use the threat of tests and the implied threat of low test grades to control student behavior. In an attempt to motivate students to prepare for and attend class, a teacher may decide to give unannounced tests; the student who is absent that day will earn a score of zero, and the student who does not do the assigned readings will likely earn a low score. This practice is unfair to students because they need sufficient time to prepare for a test in order to demonstrate their maximum performance, as discussed in chapter 3. Using tests in a punitive, threatening, or vindictive way is unethical (Nitko, 1996).

ETHICAL ISSUES

Ethical standards make it possible for nurses and patients to achieve understanding of and respect for each other (Husted & Husted, 1995); these standards also should govern the relationships of teachers and students. According to Husted and Husted, contemporary bioethical standards include those of autonomy, freedom, veracity, privacy, beneficence, and fidelity. Several of these standards are discussed here as they apply to common issues in testing and evaluation.

The standards of privacy, autonomy, and veracity relate to the ownership and security of tests and test results. Some of the questions that have been raised are: Who owns the test? Who owns the test results? Who has or should have access to the test results? and Should test-takers have access to standardized test items and their own responses?

Since educational institutions and employers started using standard-ized tests to make decisions about admission and employment, the pub-lic has been concerned about the potential discriminatory use of test results. The result of this public concern was the passage of federal and state "Truth in Testing" laws, requiring greater access to tests and test results. Some of these laws require publishers of standardized tests to sup-ply copies of the test, the answer key, and the test-taker's own responses upon request, allowing the student to verify the accuracy of the test score. Such requirements may increase the costs of testing, because test publish-ers may need to develop multiple equivalent forms of a test that has been released to students (Nitko, 1996).

Test-takers have the right to expect that certain information about them will be held in confidence. Teachers, therefore, have an obligation to main-tain a privacy standard regarding students' test scores. Access to a stu-dent's test scores and other assessment results is limited by laws such as the Family and Educational Rights and Privacy Act of 1974. Such practices as public posting of test scores and grades should be examined in light of this privacy standard. In most cases, teachers should not post assessment results if individual students' identities can be linked with their results; for this reason, many educational programs do not allow scores to be posted with student names or identification numbers. During posttest dis-cussions, teachers should not ask students to raise their hands to indicate if they answered an item correctly or incorrectly; this practice can be con-sidered invasion of students' privacy (Nitko, 1996, pp. 87, 308).

An additional privacy concern relates to the practice of keeping stu-dent records that include test scores and other assessment results. Questions often arise about who should have access to these files and the information they contain. The Family and Educational Rights and Privacy Act of 1974 limits access to a student's records to those who have legiti-mate rights to the information in order to meet the educational needs of the student. This law also specifies that a student's assessment results may not be transferred to another institution without written authorization from the student. In addition to these limits on access to student records, teachers should assure that the information in the records is accurate, and should correct errors when they are discovered. Files should be purged of anecdotal material when this information is no longer needed (Nitko, 1996, p. 87).

Another way to violate students' privacy is to share confidential infor-mation about their assessment results with other teachers. To a certain extent, a teacher should communicate information about a student's strengths and weaknesses to other teachers to help them to meet that stu-dent's learning needs. In most cases, however, this information can be communicated through student records to which other teachers have legitimate access. Informal conversations about students, especially if those conversations center on the teacher's impressions and judgments rather than verifiable data such as test scores, can be construed as gossip.

Test results sometimes are used for research and program evaluation purposes. As long as students' identities are not revealed, their scores usually can be used for these purposes (Nitko, 1996, p. 87). One way to assure that this use of test results is ethical is to announce to students when they enter an educational program that test results occasionally will be used to assess program effectiveness. Students may be asked for their informed consent for their scores to be used, or their consent may be implied by their voluntary participation in optional program evaluation activities. For example, if a questionnaire about student satisfaction with the program is distributed or mailed to students, those who wish to participate simply complete the questionnaire and return it; no written consent form is required.

Standards for Ethical Testing Practice

Several codes of ethical conduct in using tests and other assessments have been published by professional associations. These include the *Code of Professional Responsibilities in Educational Measurement* (National Council on Measurement in Education [NCME], 1995) (Appendix B); *Code of Fair Testing Practices in Education* (Joint Committee on Testing Practices, 1988) (Appendix B); and *Standards for Educational and Psychological Testing* (American Education Research Association, American Psychological Association, & NCME, 1985). Common elements of these codes and standards are discussed here.

Teachers are responsible for the quality of the tests they develop and for selecting tests that are appropriate for their intended use. Test administration procedures must be fair to all students and protect their safety, health, and welfare. Teachers are responsible for the accurate scoring of tests and reporting test results to students in a timely manner. Test results should be interpreted and used in valid ways. Teachers also must communicate test results accurately and anticipate the consequences of using results to minimize negative results to students (Nitko, 1996, pp. 79–82).

LEGAL ASPECTS

It is beyond the scope of this textbook to interpret laws that affect the use of tests and other assessments, and the authors are not qualified to give legal advice to teachers concerning their evaluation practices. However, it is appropriate to discuss a few legal issues to provide guidance to teachers in using tests.

A number of issues have been raised in the courts by students claiming violations of their rights by testing programs. These issues include race or gender discrimination, violation of due process or loss of property interests, various psychometric aspects such as the validity and reliability of tests, and accommodations for the disabled (Nitko, 1996, pp. 90–91).

Evaluation of Students with Disabilities

The Americans with Disabilities Act (ADA) of 1990 has influenced testing and evaluation practices in nursing education and employment settings. This law prohibits discrimination against qualified individuals with disabilities. A qualified individual with a disability is defined as a person with a physical or mental impairment that substantially limits major life activities. In the context of nursing education programs, qualified individuals with disabilities meet the essential requirements for participation in the program with or without accommodation or modifications (Davidson, 1994). The ADA requires teachers to make reasonable accommodations for disabled students in order to assess them properly. Such accommodations may include oral testing, computer testing, modified answer format, extended time for exams, test readers or sign language interpreters, a private testing area, or the use of large type for printed tests (Klisch, 1994; Letizia, 1995; Nitko, 1996, pp. 82-83). NCLEX policies permit test-takers with learning disabilities to have extended testing time as well as other reasonable accommodations. Persons of a cultural or racial minority, or those who speak English as a second language, however, are not considered to be persons with qualified disabilities (Klisch, 1994).

A number of concerns have been raised regarding the provision of reasonable accommodation for students with disabilities. One issue is the validity of the test result interpretations if the test was administered under standard conditions for one group of students and under accommodated conditions for other students. The privacy rights of students with disabilities is another issue; should the use of accommodated conditions be noted along with the student's test score? Such a notation would identify the student as disabled to anyone who had access to the record. There are no easy answers to such questions. In general, teachers should be guided by accommodation policies developed by each educational program and reviewed by legal counsel to ensure compliance with the ADA (Nitko, 1996, pp. 88-89).

SUMMARY

Educational testing and evaluation are growing in use and importance for society in general and nursing in particular. Nursing has come under increasing public pressure to be accountable for the quality of educational programs and the competency of its practitioners, and testing and evaluation often are used to provide evidence of quality and competence. With increasing use of evaluation and testing comes intensified interest and concern about fairness, appropriateness, and impact.

The social impact of testing can have positive and negative consequences for individuals. Tests can provide information to assist in decision making, such as selecting individuals for admission to education programs or for employment. The way in which selection decisions are made can be a matter of controversy regarding equality of opportunity and access to educational programs and jobs.

The public often expresses concerns about testing. Common criticisms of tests include: tests are biased or unfair to some groups of test-takers; test scores have little meaning because of grade inflation; testing causes emotional or psychological harm to students; and tests are used in a punitive, threatening, or vindictive way. By understanding and applying codes for the responsible and ethical use of tests, teachers can assure the proper use of assessment procedures and valid interpretation of test results. Teachers must be responsible for the quality of the tests they develop and for selecting tests that are appropriate for their intended use.

The Americans with Disabilities Act of 1990 has implications for the proper assessment of students with physical and mental disabilities. This law requires educational programs to make reasonable testing accommodations for disabled students.

REFERENCES

American Education Research Association, American Psychological Association, & National Council on Measurement in Education. (1985). *Standards for educational and psychological testing*. Washington, DC: American Psychological Association.

American Nurses Association. (1995). *Nursing's social policy statement*. Washington, DC: Author.

Americans with Disabilities Act of 1990, 42 U. S. C.A. § 12101. *et seq.* (West 1993).

Berlak, H., Newmann, F. M., Adams, E., Archbald, D. A., Burgess, T., Raven, J., & Romberg, T. A. (1992). *Toward a new science of educational testing and assessment*. Albany, NY: State University of New York.

Davidson, S. (1994). The Americans with Disabilities Act and essential functions in nursing programs. *Nurse Educator, 19* (2), 31–34.

Dowd, S. B. (1995). *Teaching in the health-related professions.* Dubuque, IA: Eastwind.

Ebel, R. L., & Frisbie, D. A. (1991). *Essentials of educational measurement* (5th ed.). Englewood Cliffs, NJ: Prentice Hall.

Family and Educational Rights and Privacy Act of 1974, 20 U. S. C. A. § 1232G (West Supp. 1997).

Hambleton, R. K. (1989). Principles and selected applications of item response theory. In R. L. Lynn (Ed.), *Educational measurement* (3rd ed., pp. 147–200). New York: American Council on Education / Macmillan.

Husted, G. L., & Husted, J. H. (1995). *Ethical decision making in nursing* (2nd ed.). St. Louis: Mosby.

Joint Committee on Testing Practices. (1988). *Code of fair testing practices in education.* Washington, DC: American Psychological Association.

Klisch, M. L. (1994). Guidelines for reducing bias in nursing examinations. *Nurse Educator, 19* (2), 35–39.

Letizia, M. (1995). Issues in the postsecondary education of learning-disabled nursing students. *Nurse Educator, 20* (5), 18–22.

Lyman, H. B. (1991). *Test scores and what they mean.* Englewood Cliffs, NJ: Prentice Hall.

McDaniel, C. (1994). Anonymous grading: An ethical teaching strategy. *Nurse Educator, 19* (5), 11–12.

National Council on Measurement in Education. (1995). *Code of responsibilities in educational measurement.* Washington, DC: Author.

Nitko, A. J. (1996). *Educational assessment of students* (2nd ed.). Englewood Cliffs, NJ: Prentice Hall.

15

Program Evaluation

P rogram evaluation is the process of judging the worth or value of an educational program. One purpose of program evaluation is to provide data on which to base decisions about the educational program. Another purpose is to provide evidence of educational effectiveness in response to internal and external demands for accountability. With competing demands for increased quality and cost containment, teachers and administrators must assume greater responsibility for systematic and ongoing program evaluation (Johnson & Olesinski, 1995). This chapter presents an overview of program evaluation models and discusses evaluation of selected program components, including curriculum, outcomes, and teaching.

PROGRAM EVALUATION MODELS

A number of models currently are used to guide program evaluation activities in schools of nursing, staff education departments, and patient education programs. These models can be described as accreditation, decision-oriented, and systems-oriented approaches (Johnson & Olesinski, 1995). Accreditation models such as those used by the National League for Nursing and the Joint Commission on Accreditation of Healthcare Organizations typically use a combination of self-study and visits to the institution by a panel of experts. Program evaluation based on an accreditation model is designed to determine whether the program meets external standards of quality. Decision-oriented models, on the other hand, usually focus on internal standards of quality, value, and efficacy. These models guide evaluation activities to provide information to decision-makers for program improvement purposes. Examples of decision-oriented approaches are the Context, Input, Process, Product (CIPP) model (Stufflebeam et al., 1971) and the evaluation plan for the University of Maryland School of Nursing as described by Waltz, Chambers, and Hechenberger (1989). Systems-oriented approaches consider the inputs, processes, and outputs of an educational program. Inputs include characteristics of program participants, such as students and teachers, and resources, such as money and time. Processes are the operations of the program, including the curriculum and instructional procedures, as well as the context or environment within which the program is implemented. Program outputs include the attainment of program objectives, participant satisfaction, cost-effectiveness, and program impact (Johnson & Olesinski, 1995).

Regardless of the specific model used, the process of program evaluation assists various audiences or stakeholders of an educational program in judging and improving its worth or value. Audiences or stakeholders are those individuals and groups who are affected directly or indirectly by the decisions made, including program planners, students, teachers, alumni, administrators, patients or clients, employers, members of the profession, and the community (Johnson & Olesinski, 1995; Staropoli & Waltz, 1978). The purpose of the program evaluation determines which audiences should be involved in generating questions or concerns to be answered or addressed. When the focus is formative, to improve the program during its implementation, the primary audiences are students, teachers, and administrators. Summative evaluation leads to decisions about whether a program should be continued, changed, or terminated; in addition to program participants, affected audiences include the public and various funding agencies (Johnson & Olesinski, 1995).

When planning a program evaluation, an important decision is whether to use an external or internal evaluator. External evaluators are thought to provide objectivity, but they may not know the program or its context well enough to be effective. An external evaluator may have limited time available to conduct the evaluation, and the expense to the program being evaluated usually is greater than if an internal evaluator is used. An internal evaluator can provide a fuller understanding of the operations and environment of the program but may be influenced by bias. The best approach may be to use an internal evaluator to carry out the evaluation plan and an external evaluator to review the results and ultimately judge the worth or value of the program (Johnson & Olesinski, 1995).

CURRICULUM EVALUATION

Traditionally, many teachers have defined program evaluation in narrow terms by focusing on the curriculum. A focus on curriculum evaluation leads to generating evaluation questions such as:

Inputs
>Are there sufficient resources to support the curriculum as planned?
>Is the planned curriculum congruent with the environment of the
>>program?

Processes
>Is the curriculum being implemented as planned?
>What barriers to curriculum implementation exist?
>Are courses optimally sequenced?
>What evidence of instructional quality exists?

Outputs
>Are students achieving curriculum objectives?
>Are employers satisfied with the competencies of graduates?

Although these evaluation questions are important, an educational program involves more than a curriculum. The success of students in meeting curriculum objectives may depend as much on the quality of the students admitted to the program or the characteristics of its faculty as it does on the sequence of courses or what instructional strategies are used. Similarly, there may be abundant evidence that graduates meet the goals of the curriculum, but those graduates may not be satisfied with the program, or may be unable to pass the NCLEX or to find employment. Former accreditation criteria that focused on program and curriculum structure often were criticized for inhibiting flexibility, creativity, and the ability of educational programs to respond to the unique needs of their environments. In an effort to ensure quality of educational programs and to increase accountability for producing competent graduates, more recent accreditation criteria reflect a heightened interest in evaluation of program outcomes (Adams, Whitlow, Stover, & Johnson, 1996).

OUTCOMES EVALUATION

The evaluation of outcomes focuses on the educational effectiveness of the program. Current accreditation criteria for nursing education programs and health care organizations support the importance of evaluating the extent to which program objectives are met as well as assessing the impact of the program on the clients served by the program. Outcomes may be specified by accrediting bodies or by the program planners and participants. For example, an accrediting body may require a program to demonstrate evidence that its graduates are able to use critical thinking in practice; the program faculty may specify the satisfaction of students, graduates, employers, and clients as another important outcome. Outcomes evaluation should include both immediate results of the program and the long-term impact and should assess both intentional and unintended effects (Bevil, 1991).

When considering whether to use teacher-made or standardized assessment tools to evaluate outcomes such as critical thinking, teachers must keep in mind the qualities of effective measurement instruments, as discussed in chapter 2. The availability of a standardized test does not ensure that teachers can make valid and reliable interpretations of the test results. Teachers must define carefully the outcome they wish to measure and design or choose instruments that are congruent with their concept of that outcome (Adams et al., 1996; Beitz, 1994).

EVALUATION OF TEACHING

One other area of evaluation involves assessing the effectiveness of the teacher. This evaluation addresses quality of teaching in the classroom and clinical setting and other dimensions of the teacher's role depending on the goals and mission of the nursing program. These other roles may include service to the nursing program, college and university, community, and profession; research; and scholarship. It is beyond the scope of this book to examine the multiple dimensions of teacher evaluation in nursing; however, a brief discussion is provided about evaluating the quality of teaching in the classroom and clinical setting.

The research in nursing education suggests five characteristics and qualities of effective teaching in nursing (Oermann, 1996):

1. knowledge of the subject matter
2. clinical competence
3. teaching skill
4. interpersonal relationships with students
5. personal characteristics.

The findings of research in nursing are consistent with studies about teacher effectiveness in other fields.

An effective teacher is an expert in the content area, has an understanding of theories and concepts relevant to nursing practice, and assists students in applying them to care of clients. Knowledge of the subject matter is not sufficient; the teacher must be able to communicate that knowledge to students. Bergman and Gaitskill (1990) reported that both faculty and students indicated that the teacher must be articulate and knowledgeable.

If teaching in the clinical setting, related characteristics reflect competence in clinical practice. Nehring (1990) found that the best teachers had expert clinical skills and judgment. The importance of clinical competence has been reported in other studies as well (Bergman & Gaitskill, 1990; Pugh, 1988; Sieh & Bell, 1994). Clinical competence includes knowledge about the practice area in which teaching occurs, from a theoretical perspective, and clinical skills. Pugh (1988) found that the best teachers showed genuine interest in students, gave immediate feedback and positive reinforcement, encouraged self-evaluation, and were able to demonstrate nursing care in the clinical setting, among other qualities.

The teacher also needs skills in teaching. These skills involve ability to:

- Identify students' learning needs;
- Plan instruction;
- Lecture effectively;
- Explain concepts and ideas clearly;
- Demonstrate procedures effectively; and
- Use sound evaluation practices.

The research suggests that the teacher's skills in clinical evaluation are important in teaching. Giving positive and useful feedback, using and sharing anecdotal notes, being fair in evaluation, having clear expectations and communicating these to students, promoting independence through evaluation, and giving constructive criticism are qualities of effective teaching reported in the research (Oermann, 1996). Sieh and Bell (1994) found that the highest ranking characteristic of an effective teacher as identified by students (N=199) in associate degree nursing programs was correcting student mistakes without belittling them. Giving suggestions for improvement and prompt feedback were important qualities identified by faculty in the study.

Another important skill of the teacher is ability to establish positive relationships with students as a group, in the classroom and clinical setting, and with students on an individual basis. Bergman and Gaitskill (1990) found that, among different characteristics of effective teaching, interpersonal relationships with the teacher were ranked as most important. These characteristics included showing confidence in students, respecting them, being honest and direct, and encouraging and supporting them.

Effective teaching also depends on the personal characteristics of the teacher. Characteristics in this area include enthusiasm, having a sense of humor, admitting mistakes and own limitations, being patient, and encouraging students to succeed (Bergman & Gaitskill, 1990; Mogan & Knox, 1987; Nehring, 1990; Pugh, 1988). Oermann (1996) concluded from a review of the research that personal characteristics of the teacher may influence teaching effectiveness.

Teaching effectiveness data are available from a variety of sources. Student evaluations are a necessary but insufficient source of information. Because students are the only participants other than the teacher who are consistently present during the teaching-learning process, they have a unique perspective of the teacher's behavior over time. Students can make valid and reliable interpretations about the teacher's use of teaching methods, fairness, interest in students, and enthusiasm for the subject. Student ratings of teaching effectiveness have several limitations. They may be affected by class size, subject area, and students' expectations of the grades they will earn in the course. Students are not able to judge competently the accuracy, depth, or scope of the teacher's knowledge. These characteristics are best judged by the teacher's peers (Gien, 1991).

Faculty colleagues may be asked to observe the teacher in the classroom, clinical practice setting, or practice laboratory and to judge the quality and appropriateness of teaching materials such as handouts, syllabus, and tests. Peer evaluation also can provide information about the effectiveness of the teacher as a member of a teaching team (Johnson, 1996). Colleague evaluations may be affected by friendships, competition, and jealousy (Gien, 1991; Hulsmeyer & Bowling, 1986). Because it would be difficult to achieve statistical evidence of reliability without multiple observations by each of several colleagues, peer evaluations should be used only for formative evaluation for the purpose of improving teaching, and not to make summative decisions regarding promotion, tenure, and salary (Gien, 1991).

Administrators usually have indirect knowledge of a teacher's effectiveness based on student and peer opinions because teachers often resist direct observation of classroom and clinical teaching by administrators (Hulsmeyer & Bowling, 1986). They are able, however, to comment on a teacher's unique contributions to the overall instructional program, such as skill in lecturing to large sections of students (Fenton, 1991).

There have been a number of studies in nursing education on developing tools for evaluating teaching effectiveness that produce valid and reliable results (Fong & McCauley, 1993; Mogan & Warbinek, 1994; Reeve,

Table 15.1 Sample Questions for Measuring Effectiveness of Clinical Teachers

Clinical teacher evaluation

Purpose: These questions are intended for use in evaluating teacher effectiveness in courses with a clinical component. The questions are to be used in conjunction with the University Student Evaluation of Teaching instrument.

Clinical teaching items

Did the teacher:

1. Encourage students to ask questions and express diverse views in the clinical setting?
2. Encourage application of theoretical knowledge in the clinical setting?
3. Provide feedback regarding student strengths and weaknesses related to clinical performance?
4. Develop positive relationships with students in the clinical setting?
5. Inform students of their professional responsibilities?
6. Facilitate student collaboration with members of health care teams?
7. Facilitate learning in the clinical setting?
8. Strive to be available in the clinical setting to assist students?
9. Was the instructor an effective clinical teacher?

1994; Zimmerman & Westfall, 1988). Sample questions for evaluating the effectiveness of the clinical teacher are found in Table 15.1.

Another approach to documenting teaching effectiveness is the use of a teaching portfolio (Fenton, 1991; Melland & Volden, 1996). The portfolio is a collection of teacher-selected materials that reflect a range of teaching activities over a period of time. There is no one format for the portfolio, since it should reflect both the purpose of the evaluation, i.e., formative or summative, and the characteristics of the teacher. A portfolio should contain artifacts related to teaching such as tests, handouts, student assignments, and instructional media, as well as the teacher's reflective commentary on the meaning of the selected items. Table 15.2 includes suggestions for content of a teaching portfolio.

Table 15.2 Suggested Content of a Teaching Portfolio

Material from the faculty member
Personal philosophy of education
Statement about teaching goals
List of courses taught
Course syllabus, sample teaching materials, sample assignments, sample tests, instructional media from one or more courses
Self-evaluation of strengths and weaknesses, including steps taken to improve teaching
An edited 10-minute videotape of a class

Material from students
Summarized student evaluations of classroom and clinical teaching with reflective interpretations of these ratings and comments on how they have been used to improve teaching
Samples of student papers, good and poor, with the teacher's written comments
Unsolicited letters from students, alumni, and clinical agency staff who work with students addressing the teacher's teaching effectiveness

Material from colleagues and administrators
Peer and administrator evaluations of teaching
Peer evaluation of teaching materials
Administrator comments on the value of the teacher's contribution to the instructional program

Adapted from Fenton, E. (1991). On getting good teachers. *Carnegie Mellon Magazine, 9*(4), 48; Melland, H. I., & Volden, C. M. (1996). Teaching portfolios for faculty evaluation. *Nurse Educator, 21*(2), 35–38.

SUMMARY

Program evaluation is the process of judging the worth or value of an educational program for the purposes of making decisions about the program or to provide evidence of its effectiveness in response to demands for accountability. A number of models can be used for program evaluation, including accreditation, decision-oriented, and systems-oriented approaches. Accreditation models are designed to determine whether a program meets external standards of quality and typically use a combination of self-study and visits to the institution by a panel of experts. Decision-oriented models usually focus on internal standards of quality, value, and efficacy to provide information for making decisions about the program. Systems-oriented approaches consider the inputs, processes or operations, and outputs or outcomes of an educational program.

The process of program evaluation assists various audiences or stakeholders of an educational program in judging its worth. Audiences or stakeholders are individuals and groups who are affected directly or indirectly by the decisions made, including program planners, students, teachers, alumni, administrators, clients, employers, members of the profession, and the public. An important decision when planning a program evaluation is whether to use an external or internal evaluator. A recommended approach is to use an internal evaluator who knows the program and its context well to carry out the evaluation plan and an unbiased external evaluator to review the results and ultimately judge the worth or value of the program.

Traditional approaches to program evaluation often focused narrowly on the curriculum, and while the curriculum is an important aspect of the program, educational effectiveness may depend as much on the quality of the students selected for the program or the characteristics of the teachers as it does on the sequence of courses or instructional strategies used. A focus on curriculum structure can inhibit the ability of an educational program to respond to the unique needs of its environment. Current accreditation criteria reflect a heightened interest in evaluating program outcomes in an effort to ensure quality and increase accountability.

One area of program evaluation involves assessing the quality of teaching in the classroom and clinical setting and other dimensions of the teacher's role depending on the goals and mission of the nursing program. Research findings suggest five characteristics and qualities of effective teaching in nursing: (a) knowledge of the subject matter, (b) clinical competence, (c) teaching skill, (d) interpersonal relationships with students, and (e) personal characteristics. Teaching effectiveness data are available from a variety of sources, including students, faculty peers, and administrators. A number of studies have been conducted to develop tools for evaluating teaching effectiveness. The use of a teaching portfolio as a way to document teaching effectiveness is another approach that allows the teacher to select and comment on items that reflect implementation of a personal philosophy of teaching.

REFERENCES

Adams, M. H., Whitlow, J. F., Stover, L. M., & Johnson, K. W. (1996). Critical thinking as an educational outcome. *Nurse Educator, 21*(3), 23–32.

Beitz, J. M. (1994). Outcomes assessment: Choosing a psychometrically sound nursing achievement test. *Nurse Educator, 19*(4), 12–17.

Bergman, K., & Gaitskill, T. (1990). Faculty and student perceptions of effective clinical teachers: An extension study. *Journal of Professional Nursing, 6,* 33–44.

Bevil, C. A. (1991). Program evaluation in nursing education: Creating a meaningful plan. In M. Garbin (Ed.), *Assessing educational outcomes: Third National Conference on Measurement and Evaluation in Nursing* (pp. 53–67). New York: National League for Nursing.

Fenton, E. (1991). On getting good teachers. *Carnegie Mellon Magazine, 9*(4), 48.

Fong, C. M., & McCauley, G. T. (1993). Measuring the nursing, teaching, and interpersonal effectiveness of clinical instructors. *Journal of Nursing Education, 32,* 325–328.

Gien, L. T. (1991). Evaluation of faculty teaching effectiveness: Toward accountability in education. *Journal of Nursing Education, 30,* 92–94.

Hulsmeyer, B. S., & Bowling, A. K. (1986). Evaluating colleagues' teaching effectiveness. *Nurse Educator, 11*(5), 19–23.

Johnson, J. H., & Olesinski, N. (1995). Program evaluation: Key to success. *JONA, 25,* 53–60.

Johnston, S. R. (1996). Evaluating the effectiveness of faculty as group members. *Nurse Educator, 21*(3), 43–49.

Melland, H. I., & Volden, C. M. (1996). Teaching portfolios for faculty evaluation. *Nurse Educator, 21*(2), 35–38.

Mogan, J., & Knox, J. E. (1987). Characteristics of "best" and "worst" clinical teachers as perceived by university nursing faculty and students. *Journal of Advanced Nursing, 12,* 331–337.

Mogan, J., & Warbinek, E. (1994). Teaching behaviours of clinical instructors: An audit instrument. *Journal of Advanced Nursing, 20,* 160–166.

Nehring, V. (1990). Nursing clinical teacher effectiveness inventory: A replication study of characteristics of "best" and "worst" clinical teachers as perceived by nursing faculty and students. *Journal of Advanced Nursing, 15,* 934–940.

Oermann, M. H. (1996). Research on teaching in the clinical setting. In K. R. Stevens (Ed.), *Review of research in nursing education* (Vol. VII, pp. 91–126). New York: National League for Nursing.

Pugh, E. J. (1988). Soliciting student input to improve clinical teaching. *Nurse Educator, 13* (5), 28–33.

Reeve, M. M. (1994). Development of an instrument to measure effectiveness of clinical instructors. *Journal of Nursing Education, 33,* 15–20.

Sieh, S., & Bell, S. (1994). Perceptions of effective clinical teachers in associate degree programs. *Journal of Nursing Education, 33,* 389–394.

Staropoli, C., & Waltz, C. (1978). *Developing and evaluating educational programs for health care providers.* Philadelphia: F. A. Davis.

Stufflebeam, D. L., Foley, W. J., Gephart, W. J. Guba, E. G. Hammond, R. L., Merriman, H. O., & Provus, M. M. (1971). *Educational evaluation and decisionmaking.* Itasca, IL: Peacock.

Waltz, C., Chambers, S., & Hechenberger, N. (1989). *Strategically planning, marketing, and evaluating nursing education and service.* New York: National League for Nursing.

Zimmerman, L., & Westfall, J. (1988). The development and validation of a scale measuring effective clinical teaching behaviors. *Journal of Nursing Education, 27,* 274–277.

16

Total Quality Management and Nursing Education

Theresa L. Carroll

Total Quality Management (TQM) is a management-driven philosophy that encourages everyone in an organization to know the mission and commit to continuously improving how the work is done to meet the expectations of the customer. The history of TQM begins with Bell Laboratories, which developed TQM as a quality-control system for the war-materials industry during World War II. TQM was subsequently adapted to rebuild Japanese industry after the war. Although the principles and practices of TQM were developed initially by U. S. industries, they did not take a prominent place in organizational development until the early 1970s, when the U. S. economy was seriously challenged in the global marketplace (Featherman & Broughton, 1993). At that time, a number of corporations such as Motorola, Westinghouse, and Chrysler adopted quality-improvement principles to transform management and production operations in factories and offices.

Since the early 1980s, this philosophy of TQM and its corollaries Total Quality Improvement (TQI) and Continuous Quality Improvement (CQI) have been adapted for use in postsecondary educational institutions and health care organizations. TQM places quality at the top of the organizational agenda, whereas TQI is the process involved in improving quality (Cornesky & McCool, 1992). Continuous Quality Improvement (CQI) stresses the dimension that this emphasis on quality is ongoing and systematic. Commitment to TQM involves careful systematic analysis of the current reality and subsequent comparison of that reality to the organization's collective vision of its future. This commitment involves defining quality in terms of the product or service that is being provided to a customer.

Inherent in TQM, TQI, and CQI is the systematic application of principles of evaluation. The practical attraction of TQM is the expectation that by using principles of TQM, TQI, and CQI, quality objectives can be achieved while containing costs. This chapter provides a brief overview of TQM and discusses application of this management strategy to higher education in general and nursing education in particular. Examples from nursing staff development also are included. For purposes of this chapter, the term TQM will be used to encompass all of the concepts represented by TQM, TQI, and CQI.

REASONS FOR TQM

Four forces have been credited with causing the TQM movement to migrate from industry into higher education. These are competition, cost, accountability, and service orientation. Whether in the public or private sector, institutions of higher education are constantly competing for declining resources. In some markets, there is blatant competition for students among institutions. Through the 1980s, tuition rose faster than the Consumer Price Index. With rising costs, both prospective students and state legislatures are demanding to know what they are getting for their education dollar. Those who support higher education are demanding increased accountability for dollars spent related to program effectiveness. Program effectiveness is measured in a variety of ways including mandatory reporting requirements, testing students, and surveying alumni and employers. Particularly in the public sector, the days of faculty being the sole source of standards for higher education are probably over. The public, via the state legislatures, demand to be involved in setting standards for quality and measuring cost-to-benefit relationships (Banta, 1993; Seymour, 1995). As hospitals and other health care organizations face cost containment challenges similar to those in higher education, the utility and value of in-house staff development similarly is being questioned.

Advocates for Total Quality Management claim that it is not just another organizational technique; it is a new way of organizational life. W. Edwards Deming, an early pioneer in TQM, called TQM the third industrial revolution—the Quality Revolution (American Association of Higher Education [AAHE], 1994). Definitions of quality vary from the work of Deming (1986), which relies on cost related to uniformity and dependability, to Juran's (1989) definition, which relates to the user's opinion of the fitness of the product, to Crosby's (1979) concern for conforming to predetermined requirements.

The environment of higher education presents strong objections to the principles, language, and methods of TQM. Faculty and administrators alike resist referring to students as customers or to the work of the academy as a business (Lozier & Teeter, 1993). Yet, few among the faculty and administration would disagree that the following questions deserve to be answered:

- Should students expect to graduate in 4 years?
- Should graduates of professional programs expect to be prepared to take and pass licensing and credentialing examinations?
- Should students be able to tell a faculty member that material in last Wednesday's class was unclear?
- Should students need to stand in line for hours to complete the registration process?

Questions being asked of staff development departments include:

- What is the appropriate content and length of orientation?
- Does every new hire need the same orientation?
- What is the most effective and efficient way to assure that all employees meet minimum competency for the jobs that they perform?
- How does staff development deliver "just in time" instruction for new tasks?

Finding answers to these questions when using TQM raises such issues as "human interrelationships, understanding of the ways that work gets done, trust or the lack thereof, and the cost in increased complexity that results from abuse by a few" (Lozier & Teeter, 1993, p. 6).

IMPLEMENTATION OF TQM

Implementation of TQM in higher education and health care organizations requires a serious commitment to involving all constituents of the organization in the process of defining the business of the organization in terms of the needs of the customer. Some of the customers of higher education include students, employers of graduates, and recipients of faculty research and service. Some of the customers of staff development include staff nurses, administration, and patients. Determining how the needs of these constituencies will be met involves identifying and articulating the values that will guide present and future action. Charting a course for the future involves developing a vision of a shared reality that encompasses decisions about the business, the customer, and values, and committing the vision to writing. Goals with quality indicators need to be articulated and stated in writing. By developing written documents, institutional leadership can continuously reinforce the mission, goals, values, and vision to faculty, staff, students, and the community (Banta, 1993).

Optimally, the initiation of TQM in an organization is a sophisticated, lengthy, and potentially costly process. However, even when resources prohibit total organizational involvement, some of the lessons of TQM can be adapted to smaller scale operations in schools, programs, departments, or divisions. Beyond the exercise of collectively defining the business, identifying the customer, and clarifying values in some written format, other useful TQM practices include developing a commitment to continuous improvement, using an adaptation of the scientific method to solve problems, decision-making based on quantitative data using specific tools for analysis, using cross-functional teams, and creating a learning organization that allows decision making to be decentralized to the lowest possible level in the institution.

Every accredited nursing program has at one time or another engaged in an internal evaluation process as part of the required self-study. There is little argument that the primary business of nursing programs is the provision of education for basic and advanced practice nursing. Some quality indicators for these programs might include numbers of students successfully completing the program compared to the number who started, NCLEX pass rate, employment rates, alumni satisfaction, employer satisfaction, and the numbers of advanced practice graduates taking and passing credentialing examinations. For programs located in institutions with missions that include research, clinical practice, service, and awarding doctoral degrees, these purposes also may become part of the business of the nursing organization. Likewise, health care organizations engage in periodic evaluations by the state and the Joint Commission on Accreditation of Health Organizations. What a commitment to TQM introduces into the program evaluation process is the need for everyone associated with the program "to adopt a quality philosophy to continuously improve on how the work is done to meet the satisfaction of the customer" (Cornesky & McCool, 1992, p. v). Ongoing, systematic evaluation becomes an integral process based on continuous monitoring of what the faculty, staff, administration or others determine are the goals and quality indicators of the nursing lecture, course, level, or program.

For example, the Plan–Do–Check–Act cycle described in Table 16.1 can be adapted to the process of teaching in the classroom, whether in higher education or a health care agency. The teacher plans the lecture content, delivers the lecture, and at the end of class asks the students to submit the

Table 16.1 Plan–Do–Check–Act (PDCA) Cycle

Plan:

Identify a process in need of improvement, analyze the problems, and develop a proposal for change that will cause some type of improvement.

Do:

Run an experiment with the proposed change.

Check:

Collect data to determine whether the experiment produced the desired change.

Act:

If the experiment is successful, implement the idea more broadly; if not, learn from the mistake and try an alternative.

Note: From G. G. Lozier & D. L. Teeter (1993). Six foundations of total quality management (p. 8). In D. J. Teeter & G. G. Lozier (Eds.)*Pursuit of quality in higher education: Case studies in Total Quality Management.* San Francisco: Jossey-Bass. Copyright © 1993 by Jossey-Bass. Reprinted with permission.

answers to three questions: What is the most important thing that you learned? What is unclear? and What should be changed to help you learn better/more easily? Feedback collected in this way allows the teacher to check the effectiveness of the session, both in terms of content and teaching strategies. For the next class period, the teacher has the opportunity to clarify content and modify teaching strategies. Modifications as simple as leaving the lights on while using the overhead projector so that students can take notes, or obtaining a microphone so that the lecturer can be heard more clearly, can improve student learning and morale.

Because limited human and other resources make it impractical to work on all problems that interfere with quality work, it is necessary to set priorities and identify key critical processes. TQM provides several useful tools for systematically collecting, analyzing, and interpreting data. Table 16.2 lists and describes the most commonly used Total Quality Improvement tools. When these tools are used by cross-functional teams, effective and efficient problem solving takes place. A cross-functional team is a group of individuals who are specially chosen to represent every aspect of the work process that is under study.

Within every institution of higher education there are critical processes such as student recruitment, admission, orientation, registration, teaching, and evaluation that are common to the organization but specific to a

Table 16.2 Total Quality Improvement Tools

Affinity Diagram
- Used to examine complex and hard-to-understand problems
- Used to build team consensus
- Results can be further analyzed by a Relations Diagram

Cause-and-Effect Diagram (Fishbone)
- Used to identify causes of a problem
- Used to draw out many ideas and/or opinions about the causes

Flow Charts
- Gives a picture of the process and the system

Force-Field Analysis
- Used when changing the system might be difficult and complex

Histogram
- A bar graph that displays information about data set and shape
- Can be used to predict the stability in the system

Nominal Group Process
- A structured process to help groups make decisions
- Useful in choosing a problem to work on
- Used to build team consensus
- Used to identify ideas and opinions about the causes of a problem

Pareto Diagram
- Bar chart that ranks data by categories
- Used to show that a few items contribute greatly to the overall problem
- Helps the team identify which processes/systems to work on

Relations Diagram
- Helps the team analyze the cause-and-effect relationships between factors of a complex issue or problem
- Directs the team to the root causes of a problem

Systematic Diagram
- Used when a broad task or goal becomes the focus of the team's work
- Often used after an Affinity Diagram and/or Relations Diagram
- Used when the task is complex or when the action plan needed to accomplish the goal is complex

Note: From R. A. Cornesky, & S. A. McCool, (1992). *Total Quality Improvement Guide for Institutions of Higher Education* (p. 4). Madison, WI: Magna. Copyright 1992 by Magna. Reprinted with permission.

discipline. For example, in one university, student registration could be denied for academic reasons, failure to meet financial obligations, or non-compliance with health requirements. The only alternative available initially to students was to travel across campus from office to office to personally investigate the reasons that they could not process their registration forms for the next semester. This university recently decentralized the registration process from the registrar's office to the individual schools, and a cross-functional team was established to decrease the length of time that undergraduate nursing students spent waiting in line while holds placed upon student records by the health service and the business office were individually investigated. The cross-functional team that was formed to analyze the registration problem included representatives from the school of nursing faculty, administration, and staff; registrar; health service; business office; and student organization. With the help of a facilitator, several 2-hour sessions were used to map the process and identify bottlenecks. One solution involved starting the registration process for nursing students 2 weeks earlier in the semester and assigning the students appointment times for individualized counseling and registration sessions. Offices that were empowered to put holds on student registration were alerted to this early schedule and could insure that records were accurate, up-to-date, and recorded in the computerized student information system.

An example of TQM applications to staff development occurred when a cross-functional team of staff nurses, nurse managers, nursing staff development instructors, and resident physicians was established to study the problem of new procedures being performed before nursing staff knew how to care for patients before, during, and after the procedure. Using the tools of TQM, it was determined that the peak time for ordering new procedures coincided with the start date for new residents. A plan was initiated to include a nursing staff development representative to explain the functions of the department and how communicating with the instructors could facilitate quality patient care in the orientation for new residents.

These examples illustrate another tenet of TQM, which is the delegation of decision making to the lowest possible level in the organization. The individuals who had the most accurate information were included not only in fact-finding, but also in crafting a solution that was acceptable to the individuals and departments that would implement and benefit from the solution. This had the effect of gaining commitment from the people responsible for implementing the decision, establishing a model for communication and future problems, and creating an attitude of interdependence and trust among the departments.

However, delegating problem solving to this level in the organization requires that individuals leading the organization have confidence that the members of the cross-functional team will act in the best interests of the organization. For cross-functional teams to work effectively, organizational leaders must provide both job-related and relationship building skills training for team members. Ideally, effective cross-functional team work is supported by development of a learning organization. "A learning organization is a place where people are continually discovering how they create their reality" (Senge, 1990, p. 13). There are five component technologies inherent in learning organizations: building a shared vision, team learning, personal mastery, mental models, and systems thinking. Building a shared vision is the capacity to hold a shared picture of the future of an organization that one hopes to create. Team learning involves studying and learning to think creatively and solve problems as a group. "Personal mastery is the discipline of continually clarifying and deepening our personal vision, of focusing energies, of developing patience, and of seeing reality objectively" (Senge, 1990, p. 7). Mental models "are deeply ingrained assumptions, generalizations, or even pictures or images that influence how we understand the world and how we take action" (Senge, 1990, p. 8). Systems thinking involves being able to see the whole picture. Systems thinking is a conceptual framework for recognizing how parts fit together to form a whole (Senge, 1990).

With cost pressures as a critical issue in both higher education and health care delivery institutions, TQM methods provide one means for continuously evaluating the effectiveness of an organization in achieving its goals. Most institutional leaders recognize that it is no longer possible to take years to identify and solve problems, revise curricula, or change a program's orientation. Total Quality Management, when diligently applied, can serve as a valuable means for keeping every department in an organization aware of when, where, and how it needs to revise, refocus, retool, or reengineer.

SUMMARY

Total Quality Management is a management-driven philosophy that encourages everyone in the organization to commit to continuously improving how the work is done to meet the expectations of the customer. TQM involves the systematic application of principles of evaluation. The present reality of the organization is systematically analyzed and compared to the organization's collective vision of its preferred future. This commitment involves defining quality in terms of the product or service that is being provided to a customer.

Forces affecting the TQM movement in higher education include competition, cost, accountability, and service orientation. Implementation of TQM in educational and health care organizations requires commitment to involving all constituents of the organization in the process of defining the business of the organization in terms of the needs of the customer. Customers of higher education include students, employers of graduates, and recipients of faculty research and service; customers of staff development include staff nurses, administration, and patients. Determining how customer needs will be met involves identifying and articulating the values that will guide present and future action, developing a vision of the preferred future, and articulating goals with quality indicators.

Although implementation of TQM can be a lengthy and costly process, some of the principles of TQM can be applied on a smaller scale, even when resources prohibit total organizational involvement. Useful TQM practices include developing a commitment to continuous improvement, using an adaptation of the scientific method to solve problems, using specific tools to collect quantitative data for decision making, using cross-functional teams, and creating a learning organization that allows decision making to be decentralized to the lowest possible level in the institution.

With the increasing economic pressures in both higher education and health care delivery institutions, TQM provides a method for continuously evaluating the effectiveness of an organization in achieving its goals.

REFERENCES

American Association of Higher Education. (1994). *A first reader for higher education.* Washington, DC: Author.

Banta, T. W. (1993). Is there hope for TQM in the academy? In D. L. Hubbard (Ed.), *Continuous Quality Improvement: Making the transition to higher education* (pp. 142–156). Maryville, MO: Prescott.

Cornesky, R. A., & McCool, S. A. (1992). *Total Quality Improvement guide for institutions of higher education.* Madison, WI: Magna

Crosby, P. B. (1979). *Quality is free.* New York: McGraw-Hill.

Deming, W. E. (1986). *Out of the crisis.* Cambridge: MIT Center for Advanced Engineering Study.

Featherman, S., & Broughton, V. (1993). Maximizing flexibility for tenured faculty position with CQI. In D. L. Hubbard (Ed.), *Continuous quality improvement: Making the transition to higher education* (pp.158–179). Maryville, MO: Prescott.

Juran, J. M. (1989). *Juran on leadership for quality: An executive handbook.* New York: Free Press.

Lozier, G., & Teeter, D. J. (1993). Six foundations of Total Quality Management. In D. J. Teeter & G. G. Lozier (Eds.), *Pursuit of quality in higher education: Case studies in Total Quality Management* (pp. 5–11). San Francisco: Jossey-Bass.

Senge, P. (1990). *The fifth discipline.* New York: Doubleday.

Seymour, D. (1995). *Once upon a campus.* Phoenix, AZ: Oryx.

Appendix A

Sample Clinical Evaluation Instruments

Sample Behaviors from Rating Scale
for Formative Evaluation

Maternal-Newborn Nursing
Mid-Term Progress Report

Name _____ Date _____

	OBJECTIVE	Yes	No	Not Obs.
1.	Applies the nursing process to the care of mothers and newborns			
	A. Assesses the individual needs of mothers and newborns			
	B. Plans care to meet the patient's needs			
	C. Implements nursing care plans			
	D. Evaluates the effectiveness of nursing care			
	E. Includes the family in planning and implementing care for the mother and newborn			
2.	Participates in health teaching for maternal-newborn patients and families			
	A. Identifies learning needs of mothers and family			
	B. Utilizes opportunities to do health teaching when giving nursing care			

Note: Not obs. = not observed.

Sample Behaviors from Same Rating Scale
for Final Evaluation

Maternal-Newborn Nursing
Clinical Performance Evaluation

Name _____ Date _____

OBJECTIVE	S	U
1. Applies the nursing process to the care of mothers and newborns		
A. Assesses the individual needs of mothers and newborns		
B. Plans care to meet the patient's needs		
C. Implements nursing care plans		
D. Evaluates the effectiveness of nursing care		
E. Includes the family in planning and implementing care for the mother and newborn		
2. Participates in health teaching for maternal-newborn patients and families		
A. Identifies learning needs of mothers and family		
B. Utilizes opportunities to do health teaching when giving nursing care		

Note: S = Satisfactory, U = Unsatisfactory.

Clinical Evaluation Instrument Using
Satisfactory-Unsatisfactory Scale

Perioperative Nursing
Clinical Performance Evaluation

Name _____ Date _____

OBJECTIVE	S	U
1. Applies principles of aseptic technique		
A. Demonstrates proper technique in scrubbing, gowning, gloving		
B. Prepares and maintains a sterile field		
C. Recognizes and reports breaks in aseptic technique		
2. Plans and implements nursing care consistent with AORN Standards and Recommended Practices for Perioperative Nursing		
A. Collects physiological and psychosocial assessment data preoperatively		
B. Identifies nursing diagnoses for the perioperative period based on assessment data		
C. Develops a plan of care based on identified nursing diagnoses and assessment data		
D. Provides nursing care according to the plan of care		
E. Evaluates the effectiveness of nursing care provided		
F. Accurately documents perioperative nursing care		
3. Provides a safe environment for the patient		
A. Assesses known allergies and previous anesthetic incidents		
B. Adheres to safety and infection control policies and procedures		
C. Prevents patient injury due to positioning, extraneous objects, or chemical, physical, or electrical hazards		
4. Prepares patient and family for discharge to home		
A. Assesses patient's and family's teaching needs		
B. Teaches patient and family using appropriate strategies based on assessed needs.		
C. Evaluates the effectiveness of patient and family teaching		
D. Identifies needs for home care referral		
5. Protects the patient's rights during the perioperative period		
A. Provides privacy throughout the perioperative period		
B. Identifies and respects the patient's cultural and spiritual beliefs		

Note: S = Satisfactory, U = Unsatisfactory.

Clinical Evaluation Instruments from ADN Program

Casper College
Department of Nursing
Clinical Evaluation Tool for Nursing 1615

Student _____ *Key:*

Instructor _____ A = Acceptable

Date(s) _____ N =Needs Improvement
Not Validated

Each clinical objective has been assigned points. If the objective is marked "2," the total number of points is awarded. If the objective is marked "1," the objective is awarded only one half the assigned points. If the objective is marked "0," no points are awarded. The points are assigned according to instructor validation (including, but not limited to, direct observation, reports of patient and/or staff, written assignments, pre- and post-conference presentations of the clinical behaviors). The total number of possible points is 50. To achieve a satisfactory rating for the clinical week the student must obtain at least 37.5 points or $^3/_4$ of the validated points.

Course/Clinical Objectives

1. Function responsibly within the limitations of the ADN student role (11 points possible)

			2	1	0	NV
	CLINICAL BEHAVIORS				A	N
a.	Assumes responsibility for own actions.					
b.	Demonstrates accountability as a student of nursing as evidenced by:					
	1.	Promptness in campus/clinical lab attendance.				
	2.	Promptness in submission of written assignments.				
	3.	Legibility of written assignments.				
	4.	Accurate spelling, grammar, and use of approved abbreviations in written assignments.				
	5.	Adherence to dress code and other college policies.				
	6.	Maintenance of confidentiality.				
c.	Seeks direction of instructor for implementation of selected nursing skills.					
d.	Participates in pre- and post-conferences.					
e.	Participates actively in campus/clinical learning experiences.					
f.	Begins to utilize established channels of communication.					
g.	Transfers knowledge from classroom to the clinical setting.					
h.	With instructor assistance, evaluates own progress and performances.					

COMMENTS:

2. Describe the concept of person (10 points possible).

				2	1	0	NV

CLINICAL BEHAVIORS		A	N
a.	Identifies deviations from normal in the 5 dimensions of the person including:		
	1. Physiological		
	2. Psychological		
	3. Sociocultural		
	4. Developmental		
	5. Spiritual		
b.	Demonstrates respect for the dignity and worth of all persons.		

COMMENTS:

3. Describe the concept of environmental stressors and the ways the person adapts to internal and external forces (5 points possible).

				2	1	0	NV

CLINICAL BEHAVIORS		A	N
a.	Identifies physiological and psychological signs of stress in self.		
b.	Identifies environmental stressors for the person within a health care setting.		
c.	Identifies patients' stressors and strengths in the 5 dimensions.		
	1. Physiological		
	2. Psychological		
	3. Sociocultural		
	4. Developmental		
	5. Spiritual		
d.	Identifies coping mechanisms used by patients in response to their health status		

COMMENTS:

4. Utilize the steps of the nursing process under the direction of the instructor (8 points possible).

				2	1	0	NV	
		CLINICAL BEHAVIORS					A	N
a.		Assessing						
	1.	Collects subjective and objective assessment data from the patient and the chart.						
	2.	Demonstrates selected assessment skills.						
	3.	Summarizes assessment data verbally and/or in writing.						
	4.	Demonstrates the organization of assessment data.						
	5.	Clusters the data and identifies gaps and inconsistencies.						
b.		Analyzing/Diagnosing						
	1.	From the NANDA list, selects a nursing diagnosis problem statement.						
	2.	Formulates a nursing diagnosis statement using the P.E.S. format with instructor assistance.						
c.		Planning						
	1.	Begins to prioritize when providing patient care.						
	2.	Develops an outcome criterion that is patient focused with instructor assistance.						
	3.	Selects nursing interventions to plan nursing care with instructor assistance.						
d.		Implementing						
	1.	Begins to use dependent, independent, and collaborative nursing interventions.						
e.		Evaluating						
	1.	Evaluates care based on outcome criteria with instructor assistance						
	2.	Verbalizes the effectiveness of nursing interventions.						

COMMENTS:

5. Safely perform technical and interpersonal skills in guided learning experiences (11 points possible).

			2	1	0	NV		
		CLINICAL BEHAVIORS					A	N
a.		Technical skills:						
	1.	Completes skills within specified time.						
	2.	Rectifies hazardous conditions within the patient environment.						
	3.	Performs basic nursing care and procedures safely, accurately, and with dexterity.						
	4.	Performs nursing skills in an organized manner.						
b.		Interpersonal skills:						
	1.	Begins to communicate with patients on a therapeutic level.						
	2.	Begins to utilize active listening and identifies own blocks to communication.						
	3.	Communicates with instructors, peers, and other members of the health care team in a professional manner.						
	4.	Begins to write concise accurate nurses' notes using acceptable terminology and abbreviations.						
	5.	Reports pertinent information related to patient care.						

COMMENTS:

6. Identify the nutritional needs of persons in states of health and illness (3 points possible).

		2	1	0	NV		
	CLINICAL BEHAVIORS					A	N
a.	Identifies clinical signs of deficiencies and excesses in nutritional status.						
b.	Calculates a person's daily energy requirement.						
c.	Calculates a person's hydration needs for a 24-hour period.						
d.	Determines nutritional adequacy of a diet.						

COMMENTS:

7. Identify the position of self and others on the health/illness continuum (2 points possible).

	2	1	0	NV

CLINICAL BEHAVIORS	A	N
a. Determines the person's understanding of his/her state of health or illness.		
b. Considers the person's health beliefs and behaviors when planning care.		

COMMENTS:

Instructor Signature _____ Date _____

Student Signature _____ Date _____

S = $^3/_4$ of all validated points
U = $< ^3/_4$ of all validated points

Progress toward meeting
course/clinical objectives _____ Absent _____hrs.
Late NCP:

Yes (   )   No (   )   N/A (   )

Copy issued to student Yes (   )   No (   )

Note: From Casper College Department of Nursing, Casper, Wyoming. Printed with permission.

Casper College Department of Nursing
Clinical Evaluation Tool for Nursing 2645

Student _____

Instructor _____

Date(s) _____

Key:

A = Acceptable

N = Needs Improvement

NV= Not Validated

Each clinical objective has been assigned points. If the objective is marked "2", the total number of points is awarded. If the objective is marked "1," the objective is awarded only one half the assigned points. If the objective is marked "0", no points are awarded. The points are assigned according to instructor validation (including, but not limited to, direct observation, reports of patient and/or staff, written assignments, pre- and post-conference presentations of the clinical behaviors). The total number of possible points is 50. To achieve a satisfactory rating for the clinical week the student must obtain at least 37.5 points or $^3/_4$ of the validated points.

Course/Clinical Objectives

1. Collaborate within the ADN role in the management of care for selected patients (10 points possible).

		2	1	0	NV	
	CLINICAL BEHAVIORS				A	N
a.	Assumes responsibility for own actions.					
b.	Participates independently in pre-and post-conferences.					
c.	Maintains confidentiality.					
d.	Adheres to Casper College Nursing Department policies and procedures.					
e.	Adheres to the policies and procedures of the clinical facility.					
f.	Practices appropriate health habits in the clinical setting.					
g.	Collaborates with instructors and others to facilitate learning.					
h.	Selects appropriate resources to facilitate learning.					
i.	Displays caring behaviors toward patients, families, peers, and others concerned with patient well-being.					
j.	Provides for patient safety.					
k.	Seeks out additional learning experiences as time permits.					
l.	Initiates referral to other resources according to perceived need.					
m.	Collaborates within the ADN role for implementation of holistic patient care.					

COMMENTS:

2. Modify nursing care based on recognition of physiological, psychological, sociocultural, developmental, and spiritual dimensions (10 points possible).

	CLINICAL BEHAVIORS	2	1	0	NV	A	N
a.	Utilizes assessment of patient's physiological/psychological needs to plan and individualize care.						
b.	Adapts nursing care based on evaluation of individual sociocultural/ethnic differences.						
c.	Identifies abnormalities of physical and/or psychological development in selected patients.						
d.	Identifies achievement or nonachievement of developmental tasks.						
e.	Adapts nursing care based on patient's physical and/or psychological development.						
f.	Adapts nursing care based on recognition of individual spiritual needs.						
g.	States the relationship between laboratory data and the clinical condition of the patient.						
h.	Applies learned principles from classroom and/or campus lab to clinical situations.						
i.	Incorporates principles from nutrition and diet therapy into the plan of care.						

COMMENTS:

3. Promote adaptation to identified stressors within the person's internal and external environment (5 points possible).

	CLINICAL BEHAVIORS	2	1	0	NV	A	N
a.	Differentiates adaptive from maladaptive behaviors in patients and/or their families which will affect the illness.						
b.	Uses identified stressors/strengths to plan positive adaptation.						
c.	Reinforces positive adaptive responses.						

COMMENTS:

4. Prioritize nursing care utilizing the nursing process for selected individuals and groups experiencing commonly recurring health problems (12 points possible).

	CLINICAL BEHAVIORS	2	1	0	NV
					A N
a.	Categorizes assessment data from a variety of sources.				
b.	Utilizes a systematic form of data collection.				
c.	Justifies gaps in the data collection.				
d.	Prioritizes selected nursing diagnoses and/or collaborative problems that are patient-centered, specific, and accurate.				
e.	States the nursing diagnoses/or collaborative problems clearly and concisely in order to provide direction for nursing interventions.				
f.	Develops outcome criteria that are patient focused and realistic.				
g.	Prioritizes standard nursing interventions that are appropriate to their respective outcome criteria.				
h.	Utilizes or revises standard nursing interventions that are appropriate to their respective outcome criteria.				
i.	Revises a teaching plan based upon perceived need.				
j.	Implements a teaching plan based on identified learning needs of selected patients.				
k.	Evaluates effectiveness of nursing interventions and initiates changes as necessary.				
l.	Revises the plan of care if the outcome criteria remain unmet.				
m.	Independently organizes time effectively.				
n.	Sets appropriate priorities independently.				

COMMENTS.

5. Integrate the safe performance of technical skills into the care of patients (8 points possible).

	CLINICAL BEHAVIORS	2	1	0	NV
					A N
a.	Demonstrates competence in performing selected technical tasks.				
b.	Incorporates nursing implications into medication administration.				
c.	Communicates data accurately, concisely, and clearly, both orally and in writing.				

COMMENTS:

6. Adapt standard nursing interventions based on effective interpersonal skills with persons and families and other members of the health team (5 points possible).

2	1	0	NV

COMMENTS:

Instructor Signature _____ Date _____

Student Signature _____ Date _____

S = $^3/_4$ of all validated points
U = < $^3/_4$ of all validated points

Progress toward meeting
course / clinical objectives _____ Absent _____ hrs.
Late NCP:

Yes ( )   No ( )   N/A ( )

Copy issued to student Yes ( )   No ( )

From Casper College Department of Nursing, Casper, Wyoming. Printed with permission.

UNIVERSITY OF VERMONT
SCHOOL OF NURSING

Clinical Evaluation - Adult Health PRNU 125-126

Student _____

Faculty _____

Clinical Location _____

Dates of experience: From _____ to _____

Number of scheduled days: C.O.D. _____ Clinical _____

Number attended by student: _____ _____

In order to pass this clinical experience, you must have accomplished all four behaviors listed below. Failure to have done one or more behaviors will result in failure for the clinical experience.

DID   DID NOT

_____ _____ 1. Came to clinical with knowledge and plans that would assure safe care.

_____ _____ 2. Provided safe care.

_____ _____ 3. Stated appropriate rationale for actions.

_____ _____ 4. Demonstrated dependability and integrity.

Pass   _____

No Pass _____

Faculty signature _____ Date _____

Student signature _____ Date _____

I. As a basis for assisting individuals, families and groups to achieve their optimum level of functioning, the student:	By the end of the rotation:
	_____ Exceeded Requirements
	_____ Met All Requirements Consistently
· Wrote thorough and accurate functional assessments (biophysical) which included data about the functions, impinging factors and logical conclusions.	_____ Met Most Requirements
· Identified how pathology impinged upon normal function as a way of justifying medical and nursing care.	_____ Did Not Meet Requirements
· Care involved actions intended to prevent alterations in functions.	
· Included post discharge planning in care.	

II. As a basis for using the nursing process as a framework for practice, the student: A. Assessment: · Obtained sufficient and accurate data from the chart. · Obtained data from the computer, cardex, and care plan. · Asked pertinent questions when obtaining report so that complete information was gained. · Monitored laboratory results and incorporated that information into plan of care. · Interpreted laboratory data accurately. · Observed patients in a systematic manner. · Did "3-minute check" within first 30 minutes of care. · Incorporated physical assessment into care routine. · Interviewed families and patients to gather accurate and sufficient data. · Utilized information from health care team members as part of data base. · Interpreted accurately the meaning of collected data. · Utilized nursing diagnosis terminology accurately to classify patient's alterations.	By the end of the rotation: ____ Exceeded Requirements ____ Met All Requirements Consistently ____ Met Most Requirements ____ Did Not Meet Requirements
B. Plan: · Set appropriate care priorities. · Established goals and plans of care for each day. · Included patient and family in planning care. · Stated patient goals in measurable patient centered terms. · Prepared plans of care that were specific and individualized to the patient. · Developed plans of care utilizing a variety of current references. · Updated care plans on computer to keep them current.	By the end of the rotation: ____ Exceeded Requirements ____ Met All Requirements Consistently ____ Met Most Requirements ____ Did Not Meet Requirements

C.	Implementation: · Organized efficient care for one patient. · Followed MCHV policies when planning and implementing care. · Organized supplies for a procedure in an efficient manner before implementing the procedure. · Performed skills correctly without coaching, after having performed the psychomotor skill with supervision and coaching. · Identified rationale for steps involved in procedures. · Informed instructor and/or coassigned nurse whenever there were any questions regarding patient care, equipment or treatments. · Problem-solved during implementation of care. · Implemented care that was consistently safe. · Monitored patient frequently and knew status at any given time. · Informed instructor about any definite or questionable deviations from the patient's normal base line. · Established priorities for care based upon patient's needs at the time. · Administered medications following MCHV policy. · Discussed patient's entire medication regimen with instructor. · Established supportive nurse-patient relationships. · Identified significant information for documentation in the medical record. · Provided time for family members to express their concerns and needs. · Included family members, when appropriate, in providing care. · Demonstrated respect for patients' bodies and belongings. · Functioned as a patient advocate.	By the end of the rotation: ____ Exceeded Requirements ____ Met All Requirements Consistently ____ Met Most Requirements ____ Did Not Meet Requirements
D.	Evaluation: · Evaluated care in terms of goals set. · Critiqued plans and care identifying areas where improvement could be made another time.	By the end of the rotation: ____ Exceeded Requirements ____ Met All Requirements Consistently ____ Met Most Requirements ____ Did Not Meet Requirements

III.	As a basis for teaching individuals, families, and groups, the student: · Incorporated teaching in the care plans. · Did incidental teaching. · Used plans that included content and process when doing preplanned teaching.	By the end of the rotation: ____ Exceeded Requirements ____ Met All Requirements Consistently ____ Met Most Requirements ____ Did Not Meet Requirements
IV.	As a basis for collaborating with health team members, consumers, and other resources, the student: · Discussed ideas and information with various members of the health care team. · Worked as a team member with peers and nurses. · Presented organized, concise information when communicating with health professionals. · Worked effectively with peers (evaluated the effect of self on others and modified behavior accordingly). · Gathered and shared essential information when getting and giving reports. · Utilized the instructor appropriately. · Used assertive communication skills when interacting.	By the end of the rotation: ____ Exceeded Requirements ____ Met All Requirements Consistently ____ Met Most Requirements ____ Did Not Meet Requirements
V.	As a basis for providing leadership in health care, the student: · Identified strengths and areas that need improvement through self-evaluation. · Functioned effectively in the student coordinator role.	By the end of the rotation: ____ Exceeded Requirements ____ Met All Requirements Consistently ____ Met Most Requirements ____ Did Not Meet Requirements
VI.	As a basis for practicing as an accountable professional, the student: · Came to clinical prepared to implement a specific plan of care. · Reviewed known procedures before clinical. · Presented pertinent patient data and appropriate plans in conference. · Submitted written assignments on time. · Arrived on time for clinical. · Maintained confidentiality with all patient information. · Wrote accurate flow sheets and notes. · Demonstrated respect when communicating with the patient or about the patient to others. · Sought out learning opportunities from other student/patient situations. · Assumed responsibility for the completion of assigned patient care. (This may have included delegation to other students of certain tasks.)	By the end of the rotation: ____ Exceeded Requirements ____ Met All Requirements Consistently ____ Met Most Requirements ____ Did Not Meet Requirements
VII.	As a basis for incorporating research into practice, the student: · Shared newly learned information in conference. · Utilized library as part of clinical preparation.	By the end of the rotation: ____ Exceeded Requirements ____ Met All Requirements Consistently ____ Met Most Requirements ____ Did Not Meet Requirements

From: University of Vermont School of Nursing, Burlington, Vermont. Reprinted with permission.

CLINICAL EVALUATION INSTRUMENT USING LETTER SYSTEM

NAME _____ DATE _____ MIDTERM GRADE _____

CLINICAL INSTRUCTOR _____ DATE _____ FINAL GRADE _____

AGENCY _____ UNIT _____ CLINICAL: 180 HOURS   CREDIT HOURS: 4

*Criteria for Clinical Evaluation:

Independent (A):   Performance is safe, accurate, proficient, coordinated, without supporting cues, focuses on client.

Supervised (B):   Performance is safe, efficient, completed within a reasonable time period, with occasional supporting cues, focuses on client.

Assisted (C):   Performance is safe, skillful in parts of behavior, frequent verbal and occasional physical directive cues in addition to supportive cues, focuses more on skill and self rather than client.

Marginal (F):   Performance is safe but not alone, unskilled and inefficient, continuous verbal and frequent physical cues, focus on skills and/or self.

* Bondy, K.N. (1983). Criterion-referenced definitions for rating scales in clinical evaluations. *Journal of Nursing Education, 22,* 376–382.

OBJECTIVES/BEHAVIORAL OUTCOME	GRADE	MIDTERM COMMENTS	GRADE	FINAL COMMENTS
I. Applies knowledge of natural and human sciences to analyze the responses of individuals experiencing alterations in health that require hospitalization.				
· Integrates knowledge of anatomy and physiology, pathology, nutrition, and pharmacology to analyze responses of adults throughout the aging process. · Identifies medical-surgical treatment modalities specific to selected problems and related needs of adults in the medical-surgical setting.				
II. Utilizes the nursing process to care for adults in the medical-surgical setting.				
· Collects data relevant to the client's health care patterns. · Develops relevant, appropriate nursing diagnoses. · Develops goals that are realistic, time framed, and measurable. · Develops a plan of care that utilizes a multidisciplinary team approach. · Implements the plan of care safely. · Evaluates the plan of care.				

OBJECTIVES/BEHAVIORAL OUTCOME	GRADE	MIDTERM COMMENTS	GRADE	FINAL COMMENTS
III. Utilizes nursing, natural, and human science theory and research findings to promote the health of adults in the medical and surgical settings.				
· Utilizes theory and research findings to develop the care plan. · Utilizes theory and research findings to provide the rationale for nursing interventions.				
IV. Demonstrates the ability to communicate effectively with clients, multi-disciplinary health team members, peers, and instructors.				
· Demonstrates effective communication techniques with clients. · Reports relevant information to staff and instructors. · Charts relevant client information systematically, clearly, concisely using correct terminology. · Writes care plans systematically, clearly, and concisely using correct terminology.				

285

OBJECTIVES/BEHAVIORAL OUTCOME	GRADE	MIDTERM COMMENTS	GRADE	FINAL COMMENTS
V. Demonstrates responsibility and accountability as a professional nursing student. · Acts within established ethical/legal parameters in providing care. · Assumes responsibility for own learning. · Is prepared for clinical practice activities. · Demonstrates clinical skills required for safe, effective delivery of care.				

STUDENT MIDTERM COMMENTS

STUDENT FINAL COMMENTS

STUDENT SIGNATURE _____

FACULTY SIGNATURE _____

STUDENT SIGNATURE _____

FACULTY SIGNATURE _____

Developed by Joanne Turka, MSN, Reprinted with permission.

WAYNE STATE UNIVERSITY   NUR 212
College of Nursing   Foundations of Nursing Care in Illness

CLINICAL EVALUATION

Total Raw Score: _____   Student's Name: _____
Letter Grade: _____   Faculty's Name: _____
                                    Population/Agency: _____
                                    Date of Experience: _____

		4	3	2	1	0	
I.	Demonstrates use of the nursing process with individuals with basic health needs.						
A.	Demonstrates use of selected physical assessment skills in collection of data.						
B.	Collects data using the patient, medical record, staff and other resources.						
C.	Demonstrates ability to correlate pathophysiology with client data.						
D.	Describes scientific rationale to explain biophysical and psychosocial data.						
E.	Describes biopsychosocial and cultural needs of individuals with basic health care needs.						
F.	Selects from an accepted list nursing diagnoses based on data.						
G.	Develops goals related to the nursing diagnosis.						
H.	Describes measurable outcome criteria related to selected client goals.						
I.	Develops an individualized plan of action to meet stated goals for individuals with basic needs.						
J.	Summarizes scientific rationale which supports the plan of action.						
K.	Carries out/implements prescribed nursing actions/care.						
	SELECTED EXAMPLES: · Accurate calculation, timely administration, and knowledge of medications.						
	· Demonstrates proper aseptic technique and use of universal precautions.						
	· Demonstrates safety with technical procedures.						

L.	Reports significant changes in patient status to clinical faculty and appropriate personnel.						
M.	Shows awareness of education needs of client with basic health care needs.						
N.	Demonstrates use of outcome criteria to measure selected goal(s).						
O.	Identifies revisions of care plan based on evaluation data.						
P.	Identifies the use of community resources in discharge planning when available.						
II.	Demonstrates accountability in care of clients with basic health care needs.						
A.	Identifies own role and responsibility as a student.						
B.	Responds to individual client needs during illness.						
C.	Provides quality care to the ill client according to professional standards.						
D.	Is accountable for own nursing practice (punctual, prepared, safe).						
	SELECTED EXAMPLES: · Is prepared for clinical assignment.						
	· Is on time.						
	· Dress is appropriate.						
	· Notifies instructor and/or agency in timely manner in case of illness or unavoidable tardiness.						
	· Reports off to appropriate staff/faculty.						
	· Provides nursing coverage when away from client area.						
	· Completes assignments on time.						
III.	Identifies own learning needs and goals.						
A.	Identifies own strengths and weaknesses.						
B.	Uses learning resources.						
IV.	Communicates effectively with clients and staff.						
A.	Demonstrates use of therapeutic techniques for interaction with ill persons.						
B.	Obtains reports accurately from staff.						
C.	Charting is clear, concise, and accurate according to patient's nursing diagnosis.						
D.	Demonstrates ability to communicate effectively with staff (physicians, nurses, etc.)						

From: Wayne State University, College of Nursing, Detroit, Michigan, Reprinted with permission.

Appendix B

Codes of Ethics in Testing and Educational Measurement

Code of Fair Testing Practices in Education

Prepared by the Joint Committee on Testing Practices

The Code of Fair Testing Practices in Education states the major obligations to test takers of professionals who develop or use educational tests. The Code is meant to apply broadly to the use of tests in education (admissions, educational assessment, educational diagnosis, and student placement). The Code is not designed to cover employment testing, licensure or certification testing, or other types of testing. Although the Code has relevance to many types of educational tests, it is directed primarily at professionally developed tests such as those sold by commercial test publishers or used in formally administered testing programs. The Code is not intended to cover tests made by individual teachers for use in their own classrooms.

The Code addresses the roles of test developers and test users separately. Test users are people who select tests, commission test development services, or make decisions on the basis of test scores. Test developers are people who actually construct tests as well as those who set policies for particular testing programs. The roles may, of course, overlap as when a state education agency commissions test development services, sets policies that control the test development process, and makes decisions on the basis of the test scores.

The Code presents standards for educational test developers and users in four areas:

A. Developing/Selecting Tests
B. Interpreting Scores
C. Striving for Fairness
D. Informing Test Takers

Organizations, institutions, and individual professionals who endorse the Code commit themselves to safeguarding the rights of test takers by following the principles listed. The Code is intended to be consistent with the relevant parts of the *Standards for Educational and Psychological Testing* (AERA, APA, NCME, 1985). However, the Code differs from the Standards in both audience and purpose. The Code is meant to be understood by the general public; it is limited to educational tests; and the primary focus is on those issues that affect the proper use of tests. The Code is not meant to add new principles over and above those in the Standards or to change the meaning of the Standards. The goal is rather to represent the spirit of a selected portion of the Standards in a way that is meaningful to test takers and/or their parents or guardians. It is the hope of the Joint Committee that the Code will also be judged to be consistent with existing codes of conduct and standards of other professional groups who use educational tests.

A. Developing/Selecting Appropriate Tests*

Test developers should provide the information that test users need to select appropriate tests.

Test Developers Should:

1. Define what each test measures and what the test should be used for. Describe the population(s) for which the test is appropriate.
2. Accurately represent the characteristics, usefulness, and limitations of tests for their intended purposes.
3. Explain relevant measurement concepts as necessary for clarity at the level of detail that is appropriate for the intended audience(s).
4. Describe the process of test development. Explain how the content and skills to be tested were selected.
5. Provide evidence that the test meets its intended purpose(s).
6. Provide either representative samples or complete copies of test questions, directions, answer sheets, manuals, and score reports to qualified users.
7. Indicate the nature of the evidence obtained concerning the appropriateness of each test for groups of different racial, ethnic, or linguistic backgrounds that are likely to be tested.
8. Identify and publish any specialized skills needed to administer each test and to interpret scores correctly.

Test users should select tests that meet the purpose for which they are to be used and that are appropriate for the intended test-taking populations.

Test Users Should:

1. First define the purpose for testing and the population to be tested. Then, select a test for that purpose and that population based on a thorough review of the available information.
2. Investigate potentially useful sources of information, in addition to test scores, to corroborate the information provided by tests.
3. Read the materials provided by test developers and avoid using tests for which unclear or incomplete information is provided.
4. Become familiar with how and when the test was developed and tried out.
5. Read independent evaluations of a test and of possible alternative measures. Look for evidence required to support the claims of test developers.
6. Examine specimen sets, disclosed tests or samples of questions, directions, answer sheets, manuals, and score reports before selecting a test.
7. Ascertain whether the test content and norms group(s) or comparison group(s) are appropriate for the intended test takers.
8. Select and use only those tests for which the skills needed to administer the test and interpret scores correctly are available.

B. Interpreting Scores

Test developers should help users interpret scores correctly.

Test Developers Should:

1. Provide timely and easily understood score reports that describe test performance clearly and accurately. Also explain the meaning and limitations of reported scores.
2. Describe the population(s) represented by any norms or comparison group(s), the dates the data were gathered, and the process used to select the samples of test takers.
3. Warn users to avoid specific, reasonably anticipated misuses of test scores.
4. Provide information that will help users follow reasonable proce-

dures for setting passing scores when it is appropriate to use such scores with the test.

5. Provide information that will help users gather evidence to show that the test is meeting its intended purpose(s).

Test users should interpret scores correctly.

Test Users Should:

1. Obtain information about the scale used for reporting scores, the characteristics of any norms or comparison group(s), and the limitations of the scores.
2. Interpret scores taking into account any major differences between the norms or comparison groups and the actual test takers. Also take into account any differences in test administration practices or familiarity with the specific questions in the test.
3. Avoid using tests for purposes not specifically recommended by the test developer unless evidence is obtained to support the intended use.
4. Explain how any passing scores were set and gather evidence to support the appropriateness of the scores.
5. Obtain evidence to help show that the test is meeting its intended purpose(s).

C. Striving for Fairness

Test developers should strive to make tests that are as fair as possible for test takers of different races, gender, ethnic backgrounds, or handicapping conditions.

Test Developers Should:

1. Review and revise test questions and related materials to avoid potentially insensitive content or language.
2. Investigate the performance of test takers of different races, gender, and ethnic backgrounds when samples of sufficient size are available. Enact procedures that help to ensure that differences in performance are related primarily to the skills under assessment rather than to irrelevant factors.
3. When feasible, make appropriately modified forms of tests or administration procedures available for test takers with handicap-

ping conditions. Warn test users of potential problems in using standard norms with modified tests or administration procedures that result in non-comparable scores.

Test users should select tests that have been developed in ways that attempt to make them as fair as possible for test takers of different races, gender, ethnic backgrounds, or handicapping conditions.

Test Users Should:

1. Evaluate the procedures used by test developers to avoid potentially insensitive content or language.
2. Review the performance of test takers of different races, gender, and ethnic backgrounds when samples of sufficient size are available. Evaluate the extent to which performance differences may have been caused by inappropriate characteristics of the test.
3. When necessary and feasible, use appropriately modified forms of tests or administration procedures for test takers with handicapping conditions. Interpret standard norms with care in the light of the modifications that were made.

D. Informing Test Takers

Under some circumstances, test developers have direct communication with test takers. Under other circumstances, test users communicate directly with test takers. Whichever group communicates directly with test takers should provide the information described below.

Test Developers or Test Users Should:

1. When a test is optional, provide test takers or their parents/ guardians with information to help them judge whether the test should be taken, or if an available alternative to the test should be used.
2. Provide test takers the information they need to be familiar with the coverage of the test, the types of question formats, the directions, and appropriate test-taking strategies. Strive to make such information equally available to all test takers.

Under some circumstances, test developers have direct control of tests and test scores. Under other circumstances, test users have such control. Whichever group has direct control of tests and test scores should take the steps described below.

Test Developers or Test Users Should:

1. Provide test takers or their parents/guardians with information about rights test takers may have to obtain copies of tests and completed answer sheets, retake tests, have tests rescored, or cancel scores.
2. Tell test takers or their parents/guardians how long scores will be kept on file and indicate to whom and under what circumstances test scores will or will not be released.
3. Describe the procedures that test takers or their parents/guardians may use to register complaints and have problems resolved.

Note: The membership of the Working Group that developed the Code of Fair Testing Practices in Education and of the Joint Committee on Testing Practices that guided the Working Group was as follows:

Theodore P. Bartell
John R. Bergan
Esther E. Diamond
Richard P. Duran
Lorraine D. Eyde
Raymond D. Fowler
John J. Fremer
  (Co-chair, JCTP and Chair,
  Code Working Group)
Edmund W. Gordon
Jo-Ida C. Hansen
James B. Lingwall
George F. Madaus
  (Co-chair, JCTP)

Kevin L. Moreland
Jo-Ellen V. Perez
Robert J. Solomon
John T. Stewart
Carol Kehr Tittle
  (Co-chair, JCTP)
Nicholas A. Vacc
Michael J. Zieky
Debra Boltas and Wayne
  Camera of the American
  Psychological Association
  served as staff liaisons

Additional copies of the Code may be obtained from the National Council on Measurement in Education, 1230 17th Street, NW, Washington, DC 20036. Single copies are free.

The Code has been developed by the Joint Committee on Testing Practices, a cooperative effort of several professional organizations, that has as its aim the advancement, in the public interest, of the quality of testing practices. The Joint Committee was initiated by the American Educational Research Association, the American Psychological Association, and the National Council on Measurement in Education. In addition to these three groups, the American Association for Counseling and Development/Association for Measurement and Evaluation in Counseling and Development, and the American Speech-Language-Hearing Association are now also sponsors of the Joint Committee.

*Many of the statements in the Code refer to the selection of existing tests. However, in customized testing programs test developers are engaged to construct new tests. In those situations, the test development process should be designed to help ensure that the completed tests will be in compliance with the Code.

This is not copyrighted material. Reproduction and dissemination are encouraged. Please cite this document as follows:

Code of Fair Testing Practices in Education (1988). Washington, DC: Joint Committee on Testing Practices. (Mailing Address: Joint Committee on Testing Practices, American Psychological Association, 1200 17th Street, NW, Washington, DC 20036.)

Note: From the National Council on Measurement in Education. Reprinted by permission.

Code of Professional Responsibilities in Educational Measurement

Prepared by the NCME Ad Hoc Committee on the
Development of a Code of Ethics:
Cynthia B. Schmeiser, ACT—Chair
Kurt F. Geisinger, State University of New York
Sharon Johnson-Lewis, Detroit Public Schools
Edward D. Roeber, Council of Chief State School Officers
William D. Schafer, University of Maryland

Preamble and General Responsibilities

As an organization dedicated to the improvement of measurement and evaluation practice in education, the National Council on Measurement in Education (NCME) has adopted this Code to promote professionally responsible practice in educational measurement. Professionally responsible practice is conduct that arises from either the professional standards of the field, general ethical principles, or both.

The purpose of the Code of Professional Responsibilities in Educational Measurement, hereinafter referred to as the Code, is to guide the conduct of NCME members who are involved in any type of assessment activity in education. NCME is also providing this Code as a public service for all individuals who are engaged in educational assessment activities in the hope that these activities will be conducted in a professionally responsible manner. Persons who engage in these activities include local educators such as classroom teachers, principals, and superintendents; professionals such as school psychologists and counselors; state and national technical, legislative, and policy staff in education; staff of research, evaluation, and testing organizations; providers of test preparation services; college and university faculty and administrators; and professionals in business and industry who design and implement educational and training programs.

This Code applies to any type of assessment that occurs as part of the educational process, including formal and informal, traditional and alternative techniques for gathering information used in making educational decisions at all levels. These techniques include, but are not limited to, large-scale assessments at the school, district, state, national, and international levels; standardized tests; observational measures; teacher-conducted assessments; assessment support materials; and other achievement, aptitude, interest, and personality measures used in and for education.

Although NCME is promulgating this Code for its members, it strongly encourages other organizations and individuals who engage in educational assessment activities to endorse and abide by the responsibilities relevant to their professions. Because the Code pertains only to uses of assessment in education, it is recognized that uses of assessments outside of educational contexts, such as for employment, certification, or licensure, may involve additional professional responsibilities beyond those detailed in this Code.

The Code is intended to serve an educational function: to inform and remind those involved in educational assessment of their obligations to uphold the integrity of the manner in which assessments are developed, used, evaluated, and marketed. Moreover, it is expected that the Code will stimulate thoughtful discussion of what constitutes professionally responsible assessment practice at all levels in education.

Section 1: Responsibilities of Those Who Develop Assessment Products and Services

Those who develop assessment products and services, such as classroom teachers and other assessment specialists, have a professional responsibility to strive to produce assessments that are of the highest quality. Persons who develop assessments have a professional responsibility to:

1.1 ensure that assessment products and services are developed to meet applicable professional, technical, and legal standards.
1.2 develop assessment products and services that are as free as possible from bias due to characteristics irrelevant to the construct being

measured, such as gender, ethnicity, race, socioeconomic status, disability, religion, age, or national origin.

1.3 plan accommodations for groups of test takers with disabilities and other special needs when developing assessments.

1.4 disclose to appropriate parties any actual or potential conflicts of interest that might influence the developers' judgment or performance.

1.5 use copyrighted materials in assessment products and services in accordance with state and federal law.

1.6 make information available to appropriate persons about the steps taken to develop and score the assessment, including up-to-date information used to support the reliability, validity, scoring and reporting processes, and other relevant characteristics of the assessment.

1.7 protect the rights of privacy of those who are assessed as part of the assessment development process.

1.8 caution users, in clear and prominent language, against the most likely misinterpretations and misuses of data that arise out of the assessment development process.

1.9 avoid false or unsubstantiated claims in test preparation and program support materials and services about an assessment or its use and interpretation.

1.10 correct any substantive inaccuracies in assessments or their support materials as soon as feasible.

1.11 develop score reports and support materials that promote the understanding of assessment results.

Section 2: Responsibilities of Those Who Market and Sell Assessment Products and Services

The marketing of assessment products and services, such as tests and other instruments, scoring services, test preparation services, consulting, and test interpretive services, should be based on information that is accurate, complete, and relevant to those considering their use. Persons who market and sell assessment products and services have a professional responsibility to:

2.1 provide accurate information to potential purchasers about assessment products and services and their recommended uses and limitations.

2.2 not knowingly withhold relevant information about assessment products and services that might affect an appropriate selection decision.

2.3 base all claims about assessment products and services on valid interpretations of publicly available information.

2.4 allow qualified users equal opportunity to purchase assessment products and services.

2.5 establish reasonable fees for assessment products and services.

2.6 communicate to potential users, in advance of any purchase or use, all applicable fees associated with assessment products and services.

2.7 strive to ensure that no individuals are denied access to opportunities because of their inability to pay the fees for assessment products and services.

2.8 establish criteria for the sale of assessment products and services, such as limiting the sale of assessment products and services to those individuals who are qualified for recommended uses and from whom proper uses and interpretations are anticipated.

2.9 inform potential users of known inappropriate uses of assessment products and services and provide recommendations about how to avoid such misuses.

2.10 maintain a current understanding about assessment products and services and their appropriate uses in education.

2.11 release information implying endorsement by users of assessment products and services only with the users' permission.

2.12 avoid making claims that assessment products and services have been endorsed by another organization unless an official endorsement has been obtained.

2.13 avoid marketing test preparation products and services that may cause individuals to receive scores that misrepresent their actual levels of attainment.

Section 3: Responsibilities of Those Who Select Assessment Products and Services

Those who select assessment products and services for use in educational settings, or help others do so, have important professional responsibilities to make sure that the assessments are appropriate for their intended use. Persons who select assessment products and services have a professional responsibility to:

3.1 conduct a thorough review and evaluation of available assessment strategies and instruments that might be valid for the intended uses.

3.2 recommend and/or select assessments based on publicly available documented evidence of their technical quality and utility rather than on insubstantial claims or statements.

3.3 disclose any associations or affiliations that they have with the authors, test publishers, or others involved with the assessments under consideration for purchase and refrain from participation if such associations might affect the objectivity of the selection process.

3.4 inform decision makers and prospective users of the appropriateness of the assessment for the intended uses, likely consequences of use, protection of examinee rights, relative costs, materials and services needed to conduct or use the assessment, and known limitations of the assessment, including potential misuses and misinterpretations of assessment information.

3.5 recommend against the use of any prospective assessment that is likely to be administered, scored, and used in an invalid manner for members of various groups in our society for reasons of race, ethnicity, gender, age, disability, language background, socioeconomic status, religion, or national origin.

3.6 comply with all security precautions that may accompany assessments being reviewed.

3.7 immediately disclose any attempts by others to exert undue influence on the assessment selection process.

3.8 avoid recommending, purchasing, or using test preparation products and services that may cause individuals to receive scores that misrepresent their actual levels of attainment.

Section 4: Responsibilities of Those Who Administer Assessments

Those who prepare individuals to take assessments and those who are directly or indirectly involved in the administration of assessments as part of the educational process, including teachers, administrators, and assessment personnel, have an important role in making sure that the assessments are administered in a fair and accurate manner. Persons who prepare others for, and those who administer, assessments have a professional responsibility to:

4.1 inform the examinees about the assessment prior to its administration, including its purposes, uses, and consequences; how the assessment information will be judged or scored; how the results will be distributed; and examinees' rights before, during, and after the assessment.

4.2 administer only those assessments for which they are qualified by education, training, licensure, or certification.

4.3 take appropriate security precautions before, during and after the administration of the assessment.

4.4 understand the procedures needed to administer the assessment prior to administration.

4.5 administer standardized assessments according to prescribed procedures and conditions and notify appropriate persons if any nonstandard or delimiting conditions occur.

4.6 not exclude any eligible student from the assessment.

4.7 avoid any conditions in the conduct of the assessment that might invalidate the results.

4.8 provide for and document all reasonable and allowable accommodations for the administration of the assessment to persons with disabilities or special needs.

4.9 provide reasonable opportunities for individuals to ask questions about the assessment procedures or directions prior to and at prescribed times during the administration of the assessment.

4.10 protect the rights to privacy and due process of those who are assessed.

4.11 avoid actions or conditions that would permit or encourage individuals or groups to receive scores that misrepresent their actual levels of attainment.

Section 5: Responsibilities of Those Who Score Assessments

The scoring of educational assessments should be conducted properly and efficiently so that the results are reported accurately and in a timely manner. Persons who score and prepare reports of assessments have a professional responsibility to:

5.1 provide complete and accurate information to users about how the assessment is scored, such as the reporting schedule, scoring process to be used, rationale for the scoring approach, technical characteristics, quality control procedures, reporting formats, and the fees, if any, for these services.

5.2 ensure the accuracy of the assessment results by conducting reasonable quality control procedures before, during, and after scoring.

5.3 minimize the effect on scoring of factors irrelevant to the purposes of the assessment.

5.4 inform users promptly of any deviation in the planned scoring and reporting service or schedule and negotiate a solution with users.

5.5 provide corrected score results to the examinee or the client as quickly as practicable should errors be found that may affect the inferences made on the basis of the scores.

5.6 protect the confidentiality of information that identifies individuals as prescribed by state and federal law.

5.7 release summary results of the assessment only to those persons entitled to such information by state or federal law or those who are designated by the party contracting for the scoring services.

5.8 establish, where feasible, a fair and reasonable process for appeal and rescoring the assessment.

Section 6: Responsibilities of Those Who Interpret, Use, and Communicate Assessment Results

The interpretation, use, and communication of assessment results should promote valid inferences and minimize invalid ones. Persons who interpret, use, and communicate assessment results have a professional responsibility to:

6.1 conduct these activities in an informed, objective, and fair manner within the context of the assessment's limitations and with an understanding of the potential consequences of use.

6.2 provide to those who receive assessment results information about the assessment, its purposes, its limitations, and its uses necessary for the proper interpretation of the results.

6.3 provide to those who receive score reports an understandable written description of all reported scores, including proper interpretations and likely misinterpretations.

6.4 communicate to appropriate audiences the results of the assessment in an understandable and timely manner, including proper interpretations and likely misinterpretations.

6.5 evaluate and communicate the adequacy and appropriateness of any norms or standards used in the interpretation of assessment results.

6.6 inform parties involved in the assessment process how assessment results may affect them.

6.7 use multiple sources and types of relevant information about persons or programs whenever possible in making educational decisions.

6.8 avoid making, and actively discourage others from making, inaccurate reports, unsubstantiated claims, inappropriate interpretations, or otherwise false and misleading statements about assessment results.

6.9 disclose to examinees and others whether and how long the results of the assessment will be kept on file, procedures for appeal and rescoring, rights examinees and others have to the assessment information, and how those rights may be exercised.

6.10 report any apparent misuses of assessment information to those responsible for the assessment process.

6.11 protect the rights to privacy of individuals and institutions involved in the assessment process.

Section 7: Responsibilities of Those Who Educate Others About Assessment

The process of educating others about educational assessment, whether as part of higher education, professional development, public policy discussions, or job training, should prepare individuals to understand and engage in sound measurement practice and to become discerning users of tests and test results. Persons who educate or inform others about assessment have a professional responsibility to:

7.1 remain competent and current in the areas in which they teach and reflect that in their instruction.

7.2 provide fair and balanced perspectives when teaching about assessment.

7.3 differentiate clearly between expressions of opinion and substantiated knowledge when educating others about any specific assessment method, product, or service.

7.4 disclose any financial interests that might be perceived to influence the evaluation of a particular assessment product or service that is the subject of instruction.

7.5 avoid administering any assessment that is not part of the evaluation of student performance in a course if the administration of that assessment is likely to harm any student.

7.6 avoid using or reporting the results of any assessment that is not part of the evaluation of student performance in a course if the use or reporting of results is likely to harm any student.

7.7 protect all secure assessments and materials used in the instructional process.

7.8 model responsible assessment practice and help those receiving instruction to learn about their professional responsibilities in educational measurement.

7.9 provide fair and balanced perspectives on assessment issues being discussed by policymakers, parents, and other citizens.

Section 8: Responsibilities of Those Who Evaluate Educational Programs and Conduct Research on Assessments.

Conducting research on or about assessments or educational programs is a key activity in helping to improve the understanding and use of assessments and educational programs. Persons who engage in the evaluation of educational programs or conduct research on assessments have a professional responsibility to:

8.1 conduct evaluation and research activities in an informed, objective, and fair manner.

8.2 disclose any associations that they have with authors, test publishers, or others involved with the assessment and refrain from participation if such associations might affect the objectivity of the research or evaluation.

8.3 preserve the security of all assessments throughout the research process as appropriate.

8.4 take appropriate steps to minimize potential sources of invalidity in the research and disclose known factors that may bias the results of the study.

8.5 present the results of research, both intended and unintended, in a fair, complete, and objective manner.

8.6 attribute completely and appropriately the work and ideas of others.

8.7 qualify the conclusions of the research within the limitations of the study.

8.8 use multiple sources of relevant information in conducting evaluation and research activities whenever possible.

8.9 comply with applicable standards for protecting the rights of participants in an evaluation or research study, including the rights to privacy and informed consent.

AFTERWORD

As stated at the outset, the purpose of the *Code of Professional Responsibilities in Educational Measurement* is to serve as a guide to the conduct of NCME members who are engaged in any type of assessment activity in education. Given the broad scope of the field of educational assessment as well as the variety of activities in which professionals may engage, it is unlikely that any code will cover the professional responsibilities involved in every situation or activity in which assessment is used in education. Ultimately, it is hoped that this Code will serve as the basis for ongoing discussions about what constitutes professionally responsible practice. Moreover, these discussions will undoubtedly identify areas of practice that need further analysis and clarification in subsequent editions of the Code. To the extent that these discussions occur, the Code will have served its purpose.

To assist in the ongoing refinement of the Code, comments on this document are most welcome. Please send your comments and inquiries to:

> Dr. William J. Russell
> Executive Officer
> National Council on
> Measurement in Education
> 1230 17th Street, NW
> Washington, DC 20036-3078

Any portion of this code may be reproduced and disseminated for educational purposes.

Index